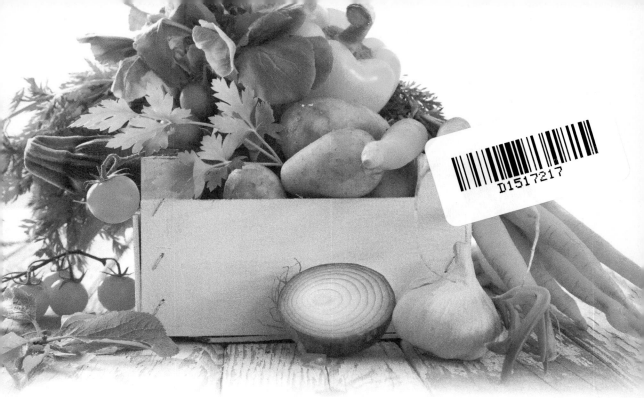

Human Nutrition
An Applied Approach

Dr. Leonard E. Gerber

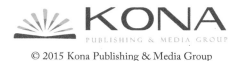

Kona Publishing and Media Group
Higher Education Division
Charlotte, North Carolina
www.konapublishing.com

Design: Rokusek Design

ISBN: 978-1-935987-67-3

Dedication

I wish to thank my entire family, living and deceased, for the encouragement they have shown in my pursuit of excellence in the field of human nutrition. In particular, a great thanks to my wife, Dr. Cynthia Jackson, for allowing me the time to write this book, and a great thanks to my late aunt, Sarah Schultz, who encouraged me and enabled me to embark on the journey that began so long ago to bring me where I am today.

Contents

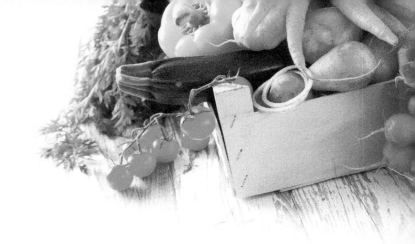

Preface

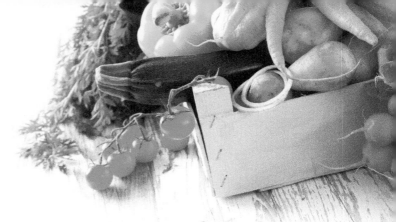

The focus of this book is to generate an awareness of the relative concerns for the various nutrients found in our diet to our overall health. Briefly, the book also dedicates some study to an awareness of the global issues in nutrition adequacy. Finally, conclusions are drawn concerning the potential directions that may be pursued to improve nutrition in the United States and abroad.

Introduction

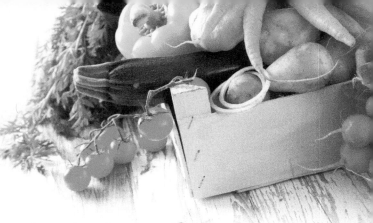

Undoubtedly, any book intended to be used as an introductory text to the science of human nutrition must provide both an understanding of the roles of the nutrients in food in human health and a perspective of the importance of these nutrients. Most texts currently available appear to do one or both of these for the reader; however, often they leave the reader with an abundance of knowledge but not information about how to apply this knowledge. I organized the current text to encourage a wider application of this knowledge, intending to foster an awareness of the relative concerns for the various nutrients found in our diet as they apply to our overall health.

Organization of This Book Compared to Other Nutrition Textbooks

The intent of this book is to initially provide some background material concerning how scientists determine nutritional needs for groups of individuals. In addition, I discuss how this advice can be applied to individuals. Also, I explore strategies that are being used and evolving toward encouraging more optimal intake of nutrients.

The individual chapters follow a pathway leading toward the reader's capacity to apply the knowledge about the nutrients. Most introductory nutrition texts are organized in a nonintegrated manner, with chapters that include a group of nutrients that are linked by a commonality in their chemistry—for instance, chapters on carbohydrates and the other energy-yielding macronutrients, chapters on micronutrients such as water-soluble vitamins, and then other chemistry-related groups. Typically chapters follow on energy balance, the various stages of the life cycle, and then topics on areas like food safety and global nutritional concerns. Other textbooks, somewhat fewer in number, choose to organize the nutrients by their roles in a specific aspect of human health. For instance, they may place nutrients in a chapter about skeletal health if one of the main functions of those nutrients relates to the skeleton's growth or maintenance. Some instructors may even use books organized by the agricultural chemistry model, and then assign sections of that book in a manner that reorganizes the material along the medical model just described.

The current book takes an approach that I believe will encourage students to be engaged with the nutrients by organizing them in a manner that is not based upon either their structural similarities or their common goals, but rather their practical significance in human diets.

Overview

Chapter 1 presents a brief introduction to the science of nutrition, including the nutrients we obtain from our diet and how they contribute to optimal function of our bodies, a general discussion of the assessment of nutritional adequacy, and the consequences of inadequacy. Chapter 2 presents current strategies that government agencies and the private sector employ to encourage a healthy diet as well as a brief description of atypical diets and the unique nutritional obstacles they present to individuals. Chapters 3 through 8 describe the roles, chemistry, and food sources of the various nutrients found in our diet, organized by their practical significance to optimal nutrition. Chapter 3 discusses required nutrients found to be most commonly inadequate in our diets. Chapter 4 follows up with those required nutrients often found inadequate due to the consumption of alternative diets or the pursuit of alternative lifestyles. Chapter 5 describes the use of food fortification and those nutrients generally found adequately in most diets due to these additions. Chapter 6 discusses those nutrients that are generally adequate but not excessive in most diets, while Chapter 7 presents concerns about those nutrients often consumed excessively in our diets. Chapter 8 focuses on those nutrients and other chemicals found in food that may have health value when consumed at levels far in excess of what we may typically consume. Chapter 9 presents recommendations for those individuals pursuing fitness activities. The final chapter presents global perspectives on diet as well as some possible solutions for domestic and global nutritional problems.

I have not included separate chapters about energy balance and weight control, nor the dietary needs of those who choose an active lifestyle, as these topics are integrated within the chapters of this book. Likewise there are no unique chapters focusing on the unique nutritional needs during the life cycle of pregnancy and lactation, infancy, childhood, adolescence, adulthood, and the senior years, as these too are integrated within the existing chapters.

The Highlights

Each chapter includes a highlight section that goes into depth concerning a topic or issue raised in the chapter. Although the chapters can be understood fully without these highlights, they can provide additional material to the interested student. I would recommend the instructor using this book assign the highlights they find important, but not necessarily discuss them within their lectures.

Aids to Student Use of This Book

The illustrations, graphs, and tables throughout the book are useful in explaining concepts often difficult to do in text form and should prove helpful to students and instructors when discussing such issues as the amounts of a nutrient found in foods or the levels of a nutrient needed by various groups of people through the life cycle. One feature found in several excellent textbooks that is replicated here is to highlight terms important to the understanding of nutrition as they first appear in the text. The word and its definition and pronunciation are then reproduced in the margin across from the term.

Suggested Readings

At the end of every chapter are reviews that interested students may find useful to further their knowledge of the topics covered in that chapter. I did not place references throughout the chapter as they often distract students and rarely are of any use to them. If any statement in this book provokes an instructor or student to require a reference source, readers can contact me at the University of Rhode Island through phone or e-mail.

The Appendices

Often these are used to provide a reference source for quantitative material or chemical structures that may interest some students. My experience is that most students don't use these types of materials. Some of these appendices are quite valuable, particularly those that include a discussion of topics providing a background in an area in which students may be weak or may want more advanced information. The appendices of this textbook include a list of useful websites and links; a discussion of digestion and absorption; a survey of nonnutritive dietary components; information on cells, genetics, and protein synthesis; and concerns about the safety of our food and water supply.

Materials Not Provided but Strongly Suggested

My classes for many years have been assigned a dietary project to assess their intake. I strongly urge that students use one of the many commercially available and reliable dietary programs for self-assessment of dietary intake.

CHAPTER

1

An Overview
of Nutritional Adequacy

My experience tells me that you are reading this book for many different reasons. Whether you are studying to be a health professional who will use nutrition as part of your skill set, are trying to learn more about an area that has attracted your personal interest, or want to learn more about an area of science that has clear personal applications, you will find this book engaging. Your instructor has selected this textbook because its intent is to allow you to see either the relationships between the **nutrients** we consume at a level beyond chemical similarities, or shared relationships with some biological or medical phenomenon.

Your food choices are important and certainly a result of many different influences. We do not have complete control over those influences, nor do we have control over the genetic influences upon our body's resistance

Nutrients: Chemical substances that supply energy or are used for maintenance, structure, or regulation.

1

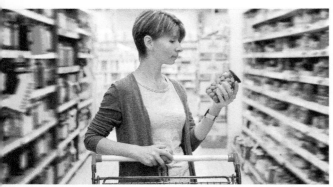

to illness. We do, however, have control over what we choose to learn and remember. The approach taken in this textbook is to prioritize your food choices based upon the nutrients typically found in the foods from which you can choose. Before you start to think about those choices, you should understand how scientists have determined the adequate levels of various nutrients for you. In addition, you should become aware of how people make food choices and what you can do to empower yourself to make choices based upon your nutritional needs.

What Nutrients Do We Obtain from Our Diet?

At the time this book is being written, scientists have identified numerous chemicals and compounds of either an **organic** or **inorganic** nature that are found in our diets. These nutrients are often divided into categories that reflect their chemical properties or structures. There are currently six classes of nutrients based upon these criteria. As mentioned before, nutrients are either organic or inorganic. The four organic categories are protein, carbohydrate, lipid (fat), and vitamins. The two inorganic categories are water and minerals.

Several other important differences exist between these categories, including whether they can be used in the body for energy as well as their essentiality. We often use the term **energy-yielding nutrients** to describe those nutrients that the body can use for energy. The term **essential nutrients** is used often to describe those nutrients that must be quantitatively available in our diets.

The compounds that are found under the category "protein" have the most in common with each other. They are always composed of the elements carbon, hydrogen, oxygen, and nitrogen. They differ structurally, however, in size and in the sequence and number of their constituent **amino acids.**

The compounds that are found under the category "carbohydrate" also have a great deal in common with each other. They are always composed of hydrogen, carbon, and oxygen. They differ between each other by the numbers of **sugars** and the types of sugars that determine their structures.

Considerable diversity is present among the compounds that are categorized as lipids or fats. Where some of the members of this group are composed primarily of various types of **fatty acids**, others are completely

Organic: A chemical substance containing either a carbon-carbon or a carbon-hydrogen bond.

Inorganic: A chemical substance containing neither a carbon-carbon or a carbon-hydrogen bond

Energy-yielding nutrient: A nutrient that can be broken down by the human body to be used for energy.

Essential nutrient: A nutrient that people must consume to maintain health as they cannot either be made at all in the body or in adequate amounts to meet needs.

Amino acids: The building blocks of protein.

Sugars: Simple carbohydrates, including monosaccharides and disaccharides.

Fatty acids: Organic compounds that have a carbon chain, with one end being an inorganic acid and the other end being a methyl group.

different and are **sterols**, the most common of which is known as *cholesterol*. There is even diversity in their elemental composition as all contain carbon, hydrogen, and oxygen but only some contain nitrogen or phosphorus.

The vitamins are the most diverse of the categories. In fact, scientists typically divide this category into two subcategories—the water-soluble vitamins and the fat-soluble vitamins—due to their striking differences in **solubility** in water versus other **solvents.**

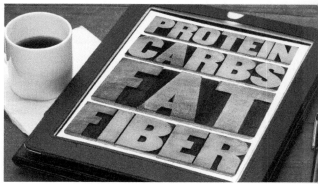

Additionally, although all vitamins are composed of carbon and hydrogen, some contain nitrogen, sulfur, cobalt, or phosphate (when activated). The differences are immense, but the fairly low levels in foods and in the body, as well as not being energy-yielding, differentiate them from the protein, carbohydrate, and lipid categories.

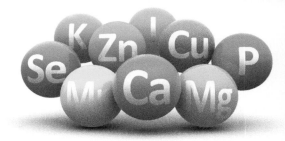

Of the two categories considered to be inorganic, water is unique in that it is composed of a collection of **molecules** that are identical to one another. In the body, water is always a liquid, as opposed to the well-known alternate forms of ice or steam that may occur in our environment.

Minerals are an extremely diverse category of inorganic materials. We are aware of about twenty-five to thirty different minerals that are in our food and water. They may be part of many different chemical structures in our food supply. The only commonality is that none of these minerals can be used as an energy source. Of course, the exception would be when carbon, hydrogen, and oxygen combine to form the carbohydrates, proteins, and lipids that for the most part are energy-yielding macronutrients.

What Nutrients Do We Need for Optimal Function of Our Bodies?

We use nutrients for a variety of purposes in our body. As discussed earlier, one significant purpose is to provide energy via the chemical breakdown of most carbohydrates, proteins, and lipids. In addition, we need nutrients for structural purposes and as components of regulatory substances in the body. Earlier the term *nutrients* was used to describe those substances found in food and used by the body. An important differentiation is the difference between nutrients and *essential nutrients*. Whereas the body uses all nutrients in some way, only the essential nutrients are required for optimal health.

Sterols: Organic compounds that have a specific four-ring carbon structure.

Solubility: The extent to which a particular chemical can be dissolved in a specific solvent.

Solvents: A liquid substance that can be used for dissolving another substance.

Molecules: Compounds consisting of one or more atoms of at least one element.

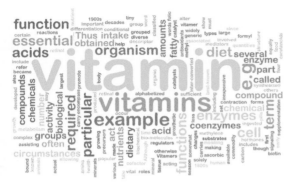

Looking back at the six categories, they can be divided into those compounds that are essential versus nonessential. For instance, protein is composed of twenty different amino acids, of which only nine are essential for healthy adult humans. Among carbohydrates, although useful to our bodies, none of them are considered essential. For lipids, we only need about a tablespoon of two types of fatty acids called *omega-3* and *omega-6* fatty acids. All but one of the thirteen vitamins are essential, as vitamin D can be produced in adequate quantities from a lipid in skin. Although research continues to determine which of the minerals is essential for human health, approximately fifteen have been determined to be essential. Of course, water is an absolutely essential nutrient and, as discussed later, will likely cause deficiency signs more quickly than any other nutrient that is dietarily inadequate.

How Do Scientists Determine the Levels of Nutrients Needed for Health?

At the current time the Food and Nutrition Board of the Institute of Medicine meets to determine what evidence is available from research studies to determine nutrient needs for various segments of the population. Recently, Canada was included with the U.S. population in making these decisions. The Food and Nutrition Board is composed of well-respected scientists in the area of food and nutrition. Although the individuals who are appointed do change, the group has been meeting since the 1940s to determine nutrient needs. After looking at all the available research regarding the needs of a particular nutrient, the board determines whether there is enough evidence to support a series of **Recommended Dietary Allowances (RDA)** for the various groups of individuals. The RDAs are calculated from the **Estimated Average Requirements (EARs)**. These numbers are determined from looking at the specific research studies that focus on the requirements for nutrients. If it is not possible to determine a requirement (RDA), but the evidence does support the nutrient being essential, then the Board will issue an **Adequate Intake (AI)** number. Energy requirements are of special concern to the board, as they do not want to encourage overconsumption of energy-yielding nutrients. As a result, all energy requirements are issued as **Estimated Energy Requirements (EERs)**, which are not increased like the EARs to statistically include the needs of 99% of the population.

Recommended Dietary Allowances (RDAs): The amount of a nutrient that has been determined to satisfy the nutritional needs of at least 98% of healthy individuals of a specific age and gender.

Estimated Average Requirements (EARs): The amount of a nutrient determined to meet the needs of healthy people of a specific age and gender.

Adequate Intake (AI): Recommended amount of a nutrient based upon the average intake of healthy people of a specific age and gender.

Estimated Energy Requirements (EERs): The amount of energy determined to meet the needs of healthy people of a specific age and gender.

The board also looks at the available evidence to determine whether a level of intake has been demonstrated to potentially cause harm when people consume more than that level. This is referred to as the **Tolerable Upper Limit (UL)**. Collectively, these standards for the various groups of individuals and the essential nutrients are called the **Dietary Recommended Intakes (DRIs)**.

Over the years, the groups and recommendations for those groups have changed. The current groups used—age, gender, and pregnancy and lactation status—are depicted in Table 1.

Tolerable Upper Intake (UL): The highest amount of a nutrient that can be safely consumed without adverse health effects for an individual of a specific age and gender.

Dietary Recommended Intakes (DRIs): Nutrient intake values used in the United States and Canada, including the EARs, RDAs, AIs, EERs, and ULs.

TABLE 1
Gender, Age, and Life Cycle Status Used in Determining RDAs

Males and Females (Age in Years)
0–0.5
0.5–1.0
1–3
4–8
9–13
14–18
19–30
31–50
>50

For Females Only
Pregnancy
1st trimester
2nd trimester
3rd trimester
Lactation
1st six months
2nd six months

What Levels of Nutrients Do We Need for Health?

Table 1 provides us with a summary of the groups for which the Food and Nutrition Board assigns Dietary Recommended Intakes but does not include the levels of the various nutrients determined to be appropriate for these groups. When discussing each nutrient, this relationship is an important part of the material covered.

How Do We Assess Nutritional Adequacy for Populations and Individuals?

Assessing Populations

Virtually all of the data used to assess nutritional adequacy is obtained from research using populations of individuals. In general, the type of research used is mostly epidemiological in nature. *Epidemiology* is the study of the relationship of an environmental influence upon disease incidence. For example, researchers in the field of psychology might survey a large population of individuals to determine the incidence of autism spectrum disorder compared to exposure to various possible toxic materials encountered in childhood. Some medical researchers might survey large groups of individuals to determine whether exposure to toxins from cigarette smoke might result in greater levels of disease such as lung cancer or cardiovascular disease. Of course, this type of research does not prove cause and effect but gives us some knowledge of an association between some environmental influence and disease incidence.

So, too, nutritional epidemiologists acquire information about whether low or high intakes of various nutrients result in disease symptoms, like a decrease in expected height or disorders of delayed development in children. In adults, nutrition researchers may look for symptoms like fatigue or weakness.

Other studies are more experimental in nature. In these studies, populations may be selected that are quite similar in age and gender and then intentionally given diets that differ in the levels of a specific nutrient. Often, subjects receive supplements in the form of a pill or capsule. Some subjects may receive a **placebo** pill or capsule with none of the nutrient contained in it. The researchers monitor some particular effect that the nutrient may have, as evidenced perhaps by the results of previous epidemiological studies. In this way, specific levels of a nutrient can be seen to affect a particular psychological or physiological characteristic. Researchers use other experimental designs that also attempt to link specific levels of a particular nutrient to an effect but are better discussed in an advanced textbook due to their more complex nature.

Placebo: A substance provided to an individual that provides no health benefit but is comparable in taste and texture to a substance that may provide a specific health benefit.

Assessing Individuals

As this book is being written, the nutritional assessment of individuals is not yet a complete reality. As the nutrients are covered throughout the chapters, students will see that while we can assess nutritional status for some nutrients, for others there is not yet the technology or knowledge to do so. For instance, the assessment of iron status can be accomplished reasonably well by noninvasive techniques but assessing the status for other minerals is not yet possible.

Nevertheless, nutritionists try to assess individuals' status to the best that current technology allows. Often, this means using statistical treatment of the DRI data that is available to determine what is appropriate for individuals. Typically, below 50% of the DRI is considered to be suboptimal, 50% to 70% of the DRI is considered to be adequate, and 70% to the Tolerable Upper Limit (UL) is considered to be a strong intake. Obviously, intake over the UL is too high since it could lead to toxic effects.

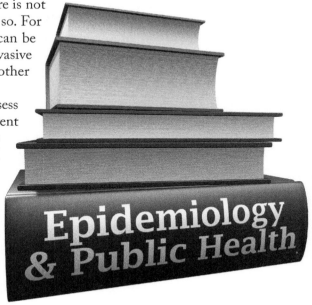

What Are the Consequences of Inappropriate Intake of Nutrients?

Suboptimal Intake

When addressing what may occur when individuals consume suboptimal intakes, some clarification is needed since nutrient requirements for individuals vary. Genetic variability as well as size of the individual can alter an individual's predicted needs. Undoubtedly the caloric needs as well as other specific nutrient needs of an extremely active individual will differ from those of a more sedentary person. Nevertheless, inadequate intake of various nutrients for all individuals can often result in deficiency symptoms. For instance, disorders like **anemia**, **osteopenia**, immune system deficiencies, cardiovascular problems, and diabetes can either be initiated or worsened.

Anemia: A reduced level of red blood cells or a reduced functionality of the red blood cells.

Adequate or Strong Intakes

Individuals consuming a nutrient at these levels will not likely exhibit either deficiency disorders or toxicity. As stated before, however, since individuals display genetic variety as well as differences in size and activity pattern, deficiency or toxicity is possible with these levels of intake.

Ostopenia: Reduction in the levels of bone compared to the normal healthy individual.

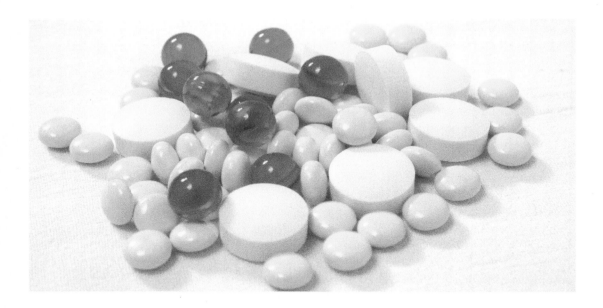

Intake above the Tolerable Upper Intake (UL)

The likelihood of toxicity occurring due to high intakes increases with the level of intake. Not all nutrients are toxic when consumed at higher levels; in addition, although some nutrients may demonstrate toxicity, their pharmacological benefits may outweigh the toxic effects. I address this phenomena later in this book.

Suggested Readings

Atkinson SA. Defining the process of Dietary Reference Intakes: Framework for the United States and Canada. *Am J Clin Nutr.* 2011; 94: 655S–657S.

Barr SI, Murphy SP, Agurs-Collins TD, Poos MI. Planning diets for individuals using the Dietary Reference Intakes. *Nutr Rev.* 2003; 61:352–60.

Murphy SP. DRIs for dietary assessment. *Asia Pac Clin Nutr.* 2008; 17, Suppl 1, 299–301.

Murphy SP, Barr SI. Challenges in using the dietary reference intakes to plan diets for groups. *Nutr Rev.* 2005; 63:267–71.

Russell RM. Current framework for DRI development: What are the pros and cons? *Nutr Rev.* 2008; 66:455–8.

Trumbo PR, Barr SI, Murphy SP, Yates AA. Dietary reference intakes: Cases of appropriate and inappropriate uses. *Nutr Rev.* 2013; 71:657–64.

HIGHLIGHT 1

Development of the National Nutrition Monitoring System

Since 1894 the U.S. government has mandated that its various divisions involved in dietary intake assessment and nutrient recommendations be actively involved in obtaining information that would lead to a better understanding of the diets of Americans.

In the beginning, the U.S. Department of Agriculture (USDA) was the sole governmental agency involved in this pursuit.

Simultaneously, as the science of medicine evolved, it became clear that governmental agencies should be involved in looking at the prevalence of certain diseases and health conditions in the U.S. population. During the 1950s, the U.S. Public Health Service was requested to investigate this relationship. The first survey, known as the National Health Examination Survey (NHES), was conducted in the early 1960s and focused upon the incidence of cardiovascular diseases, arthritis and rheumatism, and diabetes. Physical and physiological measurements were taken, such as blood pressure, serum cholesterol, skin folds, heights and weights, and electrocardiography tracings. During this decade, two additional surveys were done to evaluate disease in the population and its linkage to physical and physiological measurements.

By the end of the 1960s, it became clear that the government should link the types of medical and physiological measurements being made by the Public Health Service with the dietary data that the USDA was acquiring. As a result, the first National Health and Nutrition Exam Survey (NHANES I) was conducted from 1971 through 1974. Over 20,000 people in the United States between ages 1 and 74 were sampled for nutritional intake and status and for health and physiological assessment. The success of this survey in identifying groups of individuals whose diets may be resulting in disease occurrence resulted in two additional major surveys conducted as the NHANES II in the late 1970s and the NHANES III, which was conducted in the late 1980s through the early 1990s. The NHANES III is still being used as a significant evaluation tool, as the data was made public and those interested in statistically evaluating the data obtained can access it.

Several key issues were apparent from the results of these studies. One salient problem was the lack of adequate data for certain subgroups, like Hispanics. As a result, the Hispanic HANES was conducted to oversample this ethnic minority. Oversampling means that the researchers intentionally sampled a greater percentage of a specific group compared to the percentage they would sample in a random sampling of the overall population. In addition, those groups more likely to be at greatest nutritional risk—including those with low incomes, preschool children, and the elderly—were also oversampled.

These NHANES surveys were done with great care to sample individuals consistently. For instance, household interviews were accomplished by personnel trained to obtain demographic and socioeconomic data as well as to complete a medical history questionnaire. For the examinations, collection of samples, diagnostic tests, and dietary interviews, subjects are scheduled to meet with personnel in a mobile examination center near where they live. These mobile units travel to the area being sampled and provide a standard environment with trained personnel to collect the data that is too impractical to collect in the household setting.

The data collected during these several decades provided a great deal of information, enabling governmental agencies to assess nutritional status and risk factors that were associated with chronic diseases. Analysis of this data led directly to decisions to fortify specific foods and understand what vitamin and mineral supplements groups of individuals were consuming. Additionally, these data were extremely valuable in the initial development of food programs directed at many segments of the population.

During the time when NHANES III was undertaken, the U.S. Congress enacted legislation known as the National Nutrition Monitoring and Related Research Act of 1990. The purpose of this act was to formally link the actions of the USDA with that of the Department of Health and Human Services (HHS), formerly known as the Public Health Service. This act created the Interagency Board, which included twenty-two federal agencies with an interest in the outcome of nutrition monitoring surveys. Although many agencies benefit from the collection of nutrition information, the initial cochairs of this board were from the USDA and the HHS. Among the many responsibilities identified in this congressional act is the requirement to publish a report every five years identifying nutritional factors that likely are responsible for poor health among either the general or specific niches of the U.S. population. Rather than the original sporadic monitoring of U.S. dietary intake, the current legislation requires virtually continuous monitoring.

The development of our current monitoring system evolved from the USDA's nationwide survey of dietary intake, known as the Continuing Survey of Food Intake by Individuals (CSFII) and the NHANES, conducted by the HHS. The current integrated approach is called What We Eat in America—NHANES, which

has been in place for the last decade. The major problem with this approach has been developing and applying appropriate statistics to generalize from a small group of subjects. In addition, great discussion has taken place related as to the most appropriate way to sample daily dietary intake and consumption of dietary supplements. Significant problems have been the irregular consumption of some foods with fairly unique nutrients and the underreporting of energy-yielding macronutrients like protein.

Some of these problems are now being addressed in several ways. For instance, usual food intakes are estimated from two independent (nonconsecutive) twenty-four-hour recalls. Supplement intake is estimated from reports of dietary supplement consumption over the past month. Overreporting and underreporting both continue to be problems in estimating nutrient intakes.

One significant use of National Nutrition Monitoring has been to determine progress toward some of the national health goals identified for a particular decade set by the DHHS and assessed by the National Center for Health Statistics (NCHS). The most recent goals that we tried to meet and that have been evaluated were those identified in Healthy People 2010. In fact, we have been trying to reach goals set for each ten-year period since 1980. Unfortunately, we have often not been successful in reaching many of these goals. Although the goals are very broad, in fact there were twenty-eight focus areas in Healthy People 2010, some of them are very pertinent to the goals for optimal nutrition. The ones most relevant are found under the focus area concerning optimal weight. Additionally, some of the goals associated with optimizing food safety as well as physical activity and fitness are also important to those trying to optimize dietary practices. Currently we are striving toward the goals of Healthy People 2020, which include an additional thirteen categories. Still prominent as goals for diet are those that are under the categories of Nutrition and Weight Status as well as Food Safety and Physical Activity.

The goal for Nutrition and Weight Status is to promote health and reduce chronic disease risk through the consumption of healthful diets and achieving and maintaining healthy body weights. Americans with a healthful diet are believed to

- Consume a variety of nutrient-dense foods.
- Limit intake of saturated and trans fats, cholesterol, added sugars, salt and alcohol.

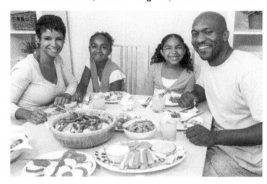

- Limit caloric intake to what is needed and avoiding unhealthy weight gain.

Perhaps we will be more successful in reaching some of these goals by the year 2020!

Suggested Readings

Barkley, GS. Factors influencing Health Behaviors in the National Health and Nutritional Examination Survey, III (NHANES III). *Social Work in Health Care.* 2008; 46:57–79.

Dwyer J, Picciano MF, Raiten DJ, et al. Estimation of usual intakes: What we eat in America—NHANES. *J Nutr.* 2003; 133:609S–623S.

Grandjean A. Dietary intake data collection: Challenges and limitations. *Nutr Rev.* 2012; 70:101S–104S.

Moshfegh A. The National Nutrition Monitoring and related research program: Progress and activities. *J Nutr.* 1994; 124:1843S–1845S.

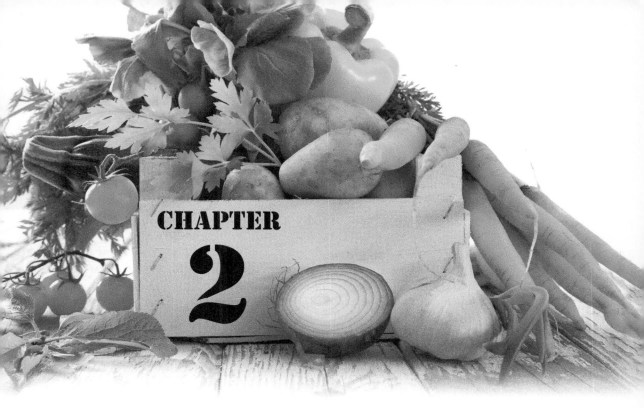

CHAPTER 2

Strategies to Maintain a Healthy Diet

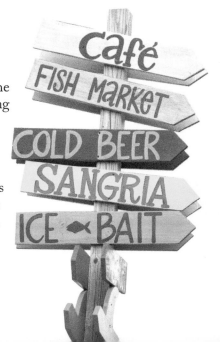

After reading the first chapter of this book and (hopefully!) the Highlight section that followed it, you should be wondering what nutritionists and dietitians are doing to encourage us to improve our diets and consequently our health. Even if you had the time to sift through all of the accumulated research on this topic, it would be difficult to draw conclusions due to the divergent opinions you would find from the true experts and the self-proclaimed experts in this field. Because those in the nutrition and dietetics field can interpret data differently, the government and the private sector each have consensus opinions about dietary plans.

Food Guides: Governmental and Private Sector

Governmental

The government has been issuing food guides since the 1940s. It is amazing how much the U.S. dietary intake has changed since then and how recommendations have changed as well. For example, when dietary guidelines were first issued, many Americans did not consume enough calories or fat. Now the problem is too much consumption of calories and fat. Likewise, substantial changes in protein and fiber consumption have taken place as well. At the end of January 2011, the USDA and the HHS jointly released the seventh edition of *Dietary Guidelines for Americans*. Although this document has many facets, one strong message is to reduce caloric intake and increase exercise. You can access the complete document by going to www.dietaryguidelines.gov for a complete listing and explanation of the guidelines. The entire document is ninety-five pages, including appendices.

Some of the other important messages aside from those associated with a reduction in obesity include

- Consuming more fruits, vegetables, and whole grains.
- Switching to low-fat and fat-free dairy products from higher-fat ones.
- Eating more seafood.
- Consuming less sodium.
- Consuming less saturated and "trans" fat.
- Consuming less added sugars and refined grains.

Because the dietary guidelines change so rapidly based upon overall food intake and exercise patterns of Americans, the Dietary Guidelines Advisory Committee, comprising fifteen experts in the field of nutrition and dietetics, have been meeting to present an updated series of recommendations for 2015.

Purpose of MyPlate

In June 2011 the Center for Nutrition Policy and Promotion issued MyPlate to replace MyPyramid, as a simpler tool to promote healthier eating than the Dietary Guidelines upon which it is based. Over the last fifty years, the simpler depiction of the Food Guide has progressed from a pie chart to a pyramid, first released in 1992 as the Food Guide Pyramid, then rereleased as MyPyramid in 2005. The current food guide, MyPlate, is available at www.ChooseMyPlate.gov, which explains its use. The current food guide is actually depicted as two plates. A large one is divided into portions corresponding to the desired amounts of fruits, vegetables, grains, or protein foods. A separate smaller plate is used to depict the relative suggested portion size for dairy foods. The design and logo for MyPlate is depicted in the margin. The key question for any of these depictions is as follows: Do they really encourage more appropriate intake of the various food groups?

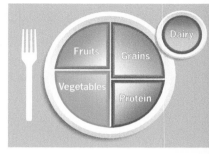

My Plate

In addition to serving as a reminder of the proportion of the food groups we should be consuming, the website provides numerous other valuable insights on proper diet and exercise. For instance, the site offers lists of preferred foods for each of the food groups, tips on preventing obesity by reducing caloric intake and increasing exercise, and tools to calculate the appropriate portions of each food group depending upon body size and other characteristics.

Criticism of MyPlate

Most of the criticism has been due to the overreliance on the MyPlate website itself to explain the information. Unless an individual has access to the Internet and an interest in using the website, MyPlate has limited value. Another critique centers on the lack of an exercise component, as was the case with MyPyramid. This oversight may lead to adherence to consumption of the food groups but a lack of concern about the necessary activity needed to prevent overweight and obesity.

Private Sector

Although the original use of the food **Exchange Lists** was to counsel people with diabetes to eat appropriately, they have become an important tool for dietitians and others to discourage overconsumption of calories. The Association of Nutrition and Dietetics, formerly known as the American Dietetics Association, presents a series of lists of foods that have similar macronutrient content and portions with similar caloric value. Each list is titled with the foods that form the majority of the entries on a particular list. There are eight lists with defined calories per serving and sometimes macronutrient levels:

Exchange lists: Groups of food organized by their carbohydrate, protein, and fat composition used as a food-planning guide that can aid in weight control.

- Vegetables: 25 calories per serving and 5 grams of carbohydrate
- Fat-free and very-low-fat milk: 90 calories per serving
- Very lean protein: 35 calories and 1 gram of fat
- Fruits: 60 calories and 15 grams of carbohydrate
- Lean protein: 55 calories and 2–3 grams of fat
- Medium-fat proteins: 75 calories and 5 grams of fat
- Starches: 80 calories and 15 grams of carbohydrate
- Fats: 45 calories and 5 grams of fat

How Do We Evaluate the Nutritional Value of Diets?

Healthy Eating Index: A method primarily developed by the USDA to evaluate the quality of diets compared to recommendations.

In general, we use the **Healthy Eating Index** to evaluate how well diets compare to the Dietary Guidelines for Americans. Although first described in 1995, the USDA updated the index in 2012 to reflect comparison with the 2010 Dietary Guidelines. The HEI-2010 has evolved from previous HEIs as goals have changed for optimal U.S. food consumption. The index is based upon scoring diets on how well they conform to what is expected from the current Dietary Guidelines. The current HEI is based upon twelve components. Nine of these components rate the diet(s) of individuals or groups on the basis of whether adequate consumption in that category was reached. Three components rate diets lower if that category is too high; they are called the *moderation components*. The current components include the following along with their rating (see Table 2).

TABLE 2
Healthy Eating Index 2010

Component	Maximum Points Adequacy
Total Fruit (includes juice)	5
Whole Fruit (excludes juice)	5
Total Vegetables	5
Greens and Beans	5
Whole Grains	10
Dairy (includes fortified soy beverages)	10
Total Protein Foods (excludes seafood and plant proteins)	5
Seafood and Plant Proteins	5
Fatty Acids (ratio of poly- and monounsaturated fatty acids to saturated fatty acids)	10
Moderation	
Refined Grains	10
Sodium	10
Empty Calories (solid fats, added sugars, and >13 grams/1000 kcal as alcohol)	20

Abridged from USDA and DHSS, Dietary Guidelines for Americans, 2010 (7th ed.). Washington, DC: U.S. Government Printing Office, 2010.

Recent uses of the HEI have been to

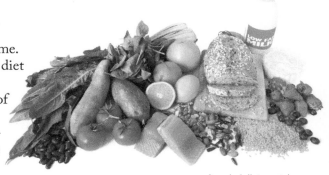

A varied diet containing many essential nutrients

- Assess changes in diet quality over time.
- Examine the relationship between diet quality and cost.
- Evaluate the quality of the diets of subpopulations.
- Evaluate the efficacy of nutrition interventions like the USDA assistance programs.

The current evaluation system is less than ideal but can provide us with at least a general idea of food consumption patterns among groups and between individuals. Clearly, other aspects of diet have an impact upon human health, but it will take time to integrate those into the guidelines and to the HEI. Highlight 2 following this chapter discusses some of the details of determining the HEI.

Atypical or Alternative Diets

The Healthy Eating Index, based upon the Dietary Guidelines, attempts to provide advice and to evaluate diets of a diverse cultural and social population. Since the components of a mixed diet are considered separately and put into the categories identified in the HEI, vegetarian, omnivore, and culturally divergent diets can be evaluated. Nevertheless, individuals can easily miss out on consumption of significant nutrients through following an atypical diet.

Vegan: An individual who refrains from consuming animal meats as well as the products of animals such as eggs and milk products.

For instance, a **vegan** can easily have inadequate intake of several nutrients due to their dietary limitations. Failure to consume any foods of animal origin eliminates poultry, red meats, fish, eggs, and dairy products. Although it is possible to still have a very high HEI with alternative food consumption, some nutrients, such as iron, vitamin B_{12}, calcium, and vitamin D, may not be consumed adequately.

Good example of vegan dietary choices

Likewise, a person who by choice or by medical necessity does not consume gluten-containing grains such as wheat can easily fail to benefit from the fortification of grain products with thiamin, riboflavin, niacin, iron, and folate.

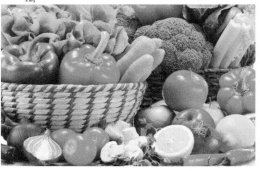

Individuals with a food allergy may also experience difficulty obtaining adequate nutrients from their diets. A common allergy is to dairy, which prevents individuals from consuming any dairy products without experiencing severe medical effects. Failure to consume foods in this category as well as the alternative of consuming fortified soy beverages is common and often results in inadequate calcium and vitamin D intake.

The above represent a few of the many alternative or atypical diets that people either consume by choice or necessity. Each alternative poses challenges for the individuals following these diets.

Nutrient Supplementation to Compensate for Dietary Deficits

Fortification

As we proceed through the various nutrients in the following chapters of this book, we will see that the U.S. government and the food industry have contributed to providing nutrients in foods that would not normally be present in them. Sometimes, this process involves adding back nutrients that are lost in the processing of foods, while at other times the nutrients added are generally not present in the foods that are receiving them.

Let's look at some examples, keeping in mind that we cover these additions in greater detail later in this book. The most striking example is the fortification of bread and other flour products with several nutrients that are lost in the milling process. For instance, while highly milled wheat flour is very low in thiamin, riboflavin, niacin, iron, and folate, whole grain and fortified products both have sufficient levels of these nutrients to provide for adequate levels in the diets of those consuming them.

Another type of fortification is to add nutrients to foods that will be good vehicles for providing these nutrients to the general public. Good examples include the addition of iodine in salt and fluoride in water, which provides adequate levels of these nutrients to people who would otherwise not receive them. Many foods are also fortified with vitamin D, such as soy beverages.

Virtually all cereals in the US are fortified with an abundance of essential nutrients.

Vitamin, Mineral, Phytochemical, and Other Supplements

Most nutrients are available in the form of pharmaceutical preparations found in various combinations. One can simply go to any pharmacy or health food store and see the plethora of different brands and combinations of nutrients for sale. Criticizing these products overall is difficult, as for some they serve a very useful purpose to maintain an adequate diet;

however only a few types of supplements are generally recommended by either the Association for Nutrition and Dietetics (AND) or the American Pediatric Association (APA). Additionally, a growing number of books from a variety of authors suggest supplement use. Most professionals in nutrition, dietetics, and medicine can agree that several risk groups certainly benefit from supplements. For instance, vegans consume diets that will likely need to be supplemented by iron, calcium, iron, vitamin B_{12}, and vitamin D. Infants may also benefit from supplements of vitamins A and D. Women during their childbearing years likely benefit from iron supple-

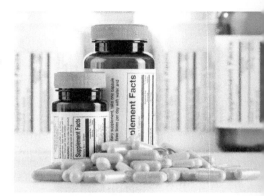

mentation. Although recently published studies have demonstrated that those who take multivitamin-multimineral supplements have a probability of having the same life span as those not taking multivitamin-multimineral supplements, the quality of life and the probability of preventing or encouraging various diseases still needs to be addressed. In particular, taking these supplements for cancer prevention needs further study, as results with respect to **initiation** and **propagation** of tumors are controversial.

Functional Foods

A recent development in the food industry has been the development of foods that either add, remove, or modify specific food components that result in health benefits. In addition, the use of natural foods containing components other than essential nutrients that improve health have been advanced. For instance, foods that are commonly consumed because their taste and texture encourage consumption are being enriched with various nutrients. This phenomenon is somewhat similar to the addition of iodine to salt or fluoride to water. Various examples are now on the market, such as margarine with omega-3 fatty acids or phytosterols. Many potato chips now have potassium added to them. Numerous foods now have fiber or **prebiotic** carbohydrates added to them.

Initiation: When referring to tumors, the initial activity that results in the start of the growth of the tumor in a single cell.

Propagation: When referring to tumors, the cellular events that result in continued growth of a tumor as many cells with the same expression.

Prebiotic: A particular food substance that enhances the growth of microorganisms in the intestine, generally referring to microorganisms that improve digestion.

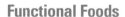

Numerous functional foods contain prebiotics

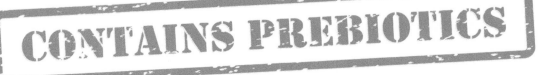

Suggested Readings

Craig WJ. Health effects of vegan diets. *Am J Clin Nutr.* 2009; 89:1627S-1633S.

Haven J, Maniscalco S, Bard S, Ciampo M. MyPlate myths debunked. *J Acad Nutr Diet.* 2014; 114: 674–5.

Mayne ST, Ferrucci LM, Cartmel B. Lessons learned from randomized clinical trials of micronutrient supplementation for cancer prevention. *Annu Rev Nutr.* 2012; 32:369–90.

Rowe S, Alexander N, Almeida N, et al. Food science challenge: Translating the dietary guidelines for Americans to bring about real behavior change. *J Food Sci.* 2011; 76:R29–R37.

Slavin JL, Lloyd B. Health benefits of fruits and vegetables. *Adv Nutr.* 2012; 3:506–16.

Watts ML, Hager MH, Toner CD, Weber JA. The art of translating nutritional science into dietary guidelines: History and evolution of the Dietary Guidelines for Americans. *Nutr Rev.* 2011; 69:404–12.

HIGHLIGHT 2

Development and Use of the Healthy Eating Index

Earlier in this chapter we discussed some uses of the Healthy Eating Index and how it was developed. In the eighteen years since it was first used, numerous changes in the Dietary Guidelines have necessitated changes in the HEI. Let's look at how those changes have evolved and the impact upon how we evaluate diets.

The original HEI was developed in 1995 by the USDA Center for Nutrition Policy and Promotion (CNPP) to measure how well the general as well as specific U.S. populations were adhering to the Dietary Guidelines for Americans. Recall that the Dietary Guidelines are the standards for appropriate diet as determined every five years since 1995 and are a collaborative effort between the U.S. Department of Agriculture (USDA) and the Department of Health and Human Services (HHS).

As originally released in 1995 the HEI had ten categories of foods that could be measured and scored to determine individual and population-based compliance with the Dietary Guidelines. Those original categories included ten components, each with a maximum score of 10 points for a total score of 100. The original HEI included the five major food groups identified at that time, four components that should be consumed in moderation, and a measure of the variety of the diet. A minimum score of 80 was considered "good," while scores between 51 and 80 indicated that improvement was needed. Scores of less than 51 were considered "poor."

Although minor changes were made to the HEI during the next decade, major changes did not occur until the release of the 2005 Dietary Guidelines, which necessitated major changes in the HEI. These newer guidelines focused more on dietary quality—in particular, whole grains vs. refined grains, the various types of vegetables, fat types vs. total fat, and "discretionary calories." This last concept is based upon the notion that individuals often consume foods that have few or no essential nutrients but the foods are caloric—for example, alcohol and candy. Researchers involved with developing these measurements tested the HEI on a large group of individuals and found that the HEI captured the adherence of individuals to the Dietary Guidelines, that the index correlated with other known measures of diet quality, and that the total possible score for the index components had a commensurate effect upon total dietary quality.

As has been set by federal law, guidelines are issued every five years; the newest Guidelines for Americans were released in 2010. Because nutrition scientists and dietitians are constantly trying to make progress as to the correct contemporary nutrition goals for the U.S. population, the new guidelines resulted in a need to produce a new HEI reflecting those goals. The new HEIs are quite complicated and sophisticated; in fact, they were not released until several years after the guidelines so that they could be sure to accurately measure compliance with the Dietary Guidelines. We discuss in detail how and why these new HEIs differ from the previous HEIs as today's diets are rated according to this system.

Although some components did not change from the previous HEIs, some components did change because of the thrust of the Dietary Guidelines. This represents both the observed changes in the U.S. diet and the level of knowledge that allows us to differentiate between the subcategories of dietary components previously not deemed to be significant.

Starting the tour of the dietary components, the first major change is the substitution of greens and beans for dark green and orange vegetables and legumes. This change reflects the current knowledge that as a nation we are furthest from our needs with respect to the vegetable subcategories of greens and beans. Orange vegetables were combined with red vegetables, with which they share numerous nutrients in common; the combined red-orange vegetables were much closer to our needs.

Total grains have been separated from whole grains, as we currently are further from our goals with respect to whole grain consumption, which provides us with numerous nutrients such as fiber, vitamins, and minerals.

With our increased knowledge of the effects of different proteins upon human health, the USDA-HHS now recommends that we replace some red meat and poultry with seafood and plant proteins. This recommendation is based upon the most current research demonstrating that vegetarian and high fish-eating diets are associated with a lower risk of cardiovascular-related risks.

Lipid researchers have actively pursued the differential effects of the various types of fatty acids upon health. As a result the Dietary Guidelines and therefore the HEIs have changed. We now believe that the type of fat is much more important than the total fat and have replaced the category of oils with a ratio of types of fatty acids consumed. The latest guidelines reflect research demonstrating that a greater amount of monounsaturated fatty acids plus polyunsaturated acids as a ratio to saturated fatty acids is a good predictor of risk reduction for cardiovascular disease. The absolute levels of saturated fat do not seem to be that significant as a predictor for disease, so that measure has also been dropped from the list of HEIs that should be consumed in moderation.

Refined grains, however, have been added as a new category in the moderation group. The rationale for this decision came from the knowledge that foods with high levels of refined grains are also often high in solid fats and added sugars.

Last, empty calories replaces the category of calories from solid fats, added sugars, and alcohol. Essentially this is primarily a name change to reflect the reality of the category, rather than using an acronym, SoFAAS, as was the case in 2005.

As mentioned in chapter 2, these HEI scores are valuable for assessing the progress of the nation and subpopulations as well. As we progress in our knowledge of nutrition and dietetics, future Dietary Guidelines will result in improved HEI scoring systems.

Suggested Readings

Guenther PM, Casavale KO, Reedy J, et al. Update of the Healthy Eating Index: HEI–2010. *J Acad Nutr Diet.* 2013; 113:569–80.

Guenther PM, Reedy J, Krebs-Smith SM, et al. Development and evaluation of the Healthy Eating Index–2005: Technical Report. Available at http://www.cnpp. usda.gov/HealthyEatingIndex.htm_

Required Nutrients Found to Be Most Commonly Inadequate in Diets

As stated earlier in this book, the organization of the chapters is based upon factors other than the typical chemistry of the nutrients, but instead upon the commonality of nutrients in typical diets, nutrients available in the diet to fortification, nutrients commonly available naturally in the diet, nutrients with potential serious toxicity and other distinctive determinants. Here we explore nutrients from different chemical categories that are often found inadequately in many diets.

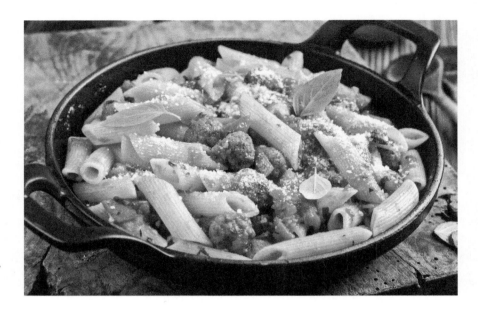

An entrée with many energy-yielding nutrients

Macronutrients

Those nutrients that can provide energy to the body because they can be broken down and result in the capture of energy for the maintenance, movement, and sometimes growth of the body are considered energy-yielding macronutrients. Often some of these nutrients possess duality and not only provide energy but are important for other physiological purposes. The two nutrients in this category that are often inadequate in typical U.S. diets are fiber and omega-3 fatty acids.

Fiber is often found in a variety of fruits, vegetables, and whole grains. Dietary fiber includes those nondigestible carbohydrates and the hydrocarbon lignin that are found in plants. More recently, functional fiber has also been included in this category, which includes those nondigestible carbohydrates that are isolated, manufactured, or extracted and may also be beneficial to humans. Another contemporary way of dividing fiber is to simply look at whether these indigestible materials are soluble in warm water. Typically those fibers that are soluble in water also form gels and can be fermented by bacteria in our lower gut. These generally include such fibers as the pectins of fruit and psyllium, a common ingredient in Metamucil®. Unfortunately, consumption of these foods is currently inadequate to provide the necessary fiber. Although recommendations for fiber intake are available from different sources, the Dietary Guidelines for Americans recommends consumption of 14 grams of fiber per 1000 kcal

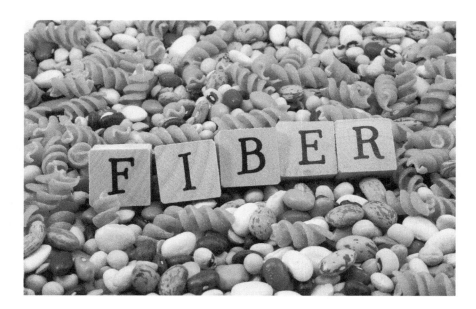

of food energy intake. The Food and Nutrition Board is more specific and recommends Adequate Intakes (AIs) for dietary plus functional fiber for individuals by age and gender. The highest levels of 38 g/d are recommended for men between the ages of 19 and 50 and for boys ages 14 to 18, while the lowest level of 19 g/d is recommended for both boys and girls from ages 1 to 3 years. The average American has an intake of about 15 g of fiber each day, which is obviously inadequate even for the group requiring the smallest amount of fiber as cited above.

So, what are the ramifications of this dietary inadequacy? At this time, scientific information demonstrates significant claims for reducing both mortality and disease through the consumption of adequate amounts of fiber. For instance, research has shown that soluble and insoluble fibers reduce the risk for heart disease, obesity, and gastrointestinal disorders including **diverticulitis,** constipation, and colon cancer. Other research has shown that soluble fibers may improve glycemic index and reduce the development of diabetes.

At this time, assigning levels of intake for specific fibers or even fiber types is impossible. Consequently, a wide variety of fiber-containing foods including whole grain cereals and breads, legumes, fruits, and vegetables is recommended. Hopefully, adherence to a diet incorporating these foods will result in adequacy of total fiber and the various types that contribute to disease reduction.

Diverticulitis: An infection of the colon, generally attributed to weak muscle walls, resulting in diverticulosis, followed by microorganisms entering the weakened areas, resulting in the infection.

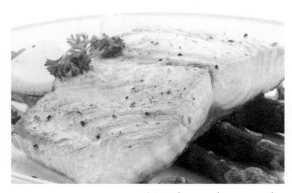

An excellent source of omega-3 fatty acids

Omega-3 fatty acids are often in short supply in U.S. diets. Despite our high consumption of fat—30% to 35% of calories consumed—we still do not consume enough of this particular type of fat. Although humans and animals can make many different types of fats from a variety of precursors, the ability to make this particular type of fat as well as the omega-6 fatty acids does not exist for us or for animals—making these two types of fats essential in our diet. For omega-6 intake, we have an abundance of plants that can produce it, so simply consuming corn oil or generic vegetable oil will suffice. It would seem that our best sources for omega-3 fats that we have are the plants in our water systems and the animals that consume those plants. Some terrestrial plants produce omega-3 fats, but research has shown that the conversion of these precursors to the more active forms that the animal body requires is likely inadequate. Most of us need to eat fish in our diet. Not all fish, however, have the same levels of omega-3 fatty acids. We should choose wisely from among those fish with higher levels, including herring, salmon, and tuna.

Why are omega-3 fatty acids important for our health? Research indicates that numerous materials are made from both omega-3 and omega-6 fatty acids. Most of these materials are the **eicosanoids**. These **hormone**-like substances can have tremendous impact upon our physiological functions; some may be injurious and some helpful. Some of the substances

Eicosanoids: Biologically active molecules produced in the body from polyunsaturated fatty acids.

Hormone: A biologically active molecule produced in one part of the body that effects the activity of other cells or organs. Often, hormonelike molecules produced in the body may affect cells or organs in close proximity to the site of production.

Molecular structures of the two most significant omega-3 fatty acids found in our diet

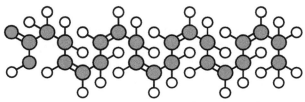

Docosahexaenoic acid (Omega-3)

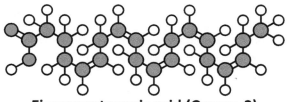

Eicosapentaenoic acid (Omega-3)

made from the omega-6 fatty acids may be associated with poor health outcomes, such as encouragement of cardiovascular disease, while the omega-3 fatty acids appear to contribute to physiological effects that reduce the probability of cardiovascular disease. Specifically, the eicosanoids made from omega-3 fatty acids lower blood pressure, prevent blood clot formation, reduce **arrhythmias**, and reduce inflammation. These activities are easily contrasted with the effects of omega-6 fatty acids, which increase inflammation, constrict blood vessels, and increase the tendency toward arrhythmias. Researchers and clinicians believe that the two types of essential fatty acids identified above must be balanced in the diet for the body to function optimally. In fact recent evidence shows that omega-6 fatty acids also protect the heart by encouraging better use of insulin and reducing the **lipoprotein** particle **LDL**, which carries cholesterol to arteries and is believed to participate in the development of cardiovascular disease.

In conclusion, although some individuals take fish oil capsules or more recently krill oil capsules, the overall benefits of fish consumption are far more significant.

Vitamins

Vitamins are organic nutrients required in small amounts in the diet to promote health. Despite numerous controversies over the last several decades about the amount of specific vitamins required, one vitamin, vitamin D, stands out as not being consumed in adequate levels in contemporary diets in the United States even though it is a fortified component in milk. Many vitamins have been added by legislative authority to flour and other grain products as well as in breakfast cereals. Although they are usually not found adequate in diets devoid of fortified foods, because most people receive adequate levels, these vitamins are discussed in a subsequent chapter focusing upon these fortified nutrients. One B vitamin, however, still stands out as being potentially a problem in the U.S. diet: B_6.

Vitamin D is the subject of much controversy among nutrition experts due to several factors, including the body's ability to synthesize vitamin D, the limited amount of foods that contain it, and changes occurring with the aging process that may alter requirements. First, let's discuss the issue of body synthesis and use. Derivatives of cholesterol, a common nonessential molecule found in the body, are found in the skin.

Arrhythmias: A variety of disorders associated with the contractility of the heart, resulting in a beating pattern that is not associated with the normal action of the heart muscle. Often these take the form of irregularity of contractions or contractions that occur more rapidly than normal.

Lipoprotein: A variety of different particles that are produced in the body that transport lipids, which also have specific proteins as part of them that result in either enhanced targeting of the lipoprotein to various tissues or organs or enhanced enzymatic activity associated with fat metabolism at a specific tissue or organ.

LDL: The abbreviation for a lipoprotein particle, known as low-density lipoprotein, whose function is to bring cholesterol to various sites in the body to be used or deposited.

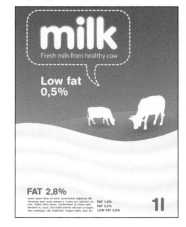

Low-fat milk consumption is an excellent way to get adequate vitamin D in your diet

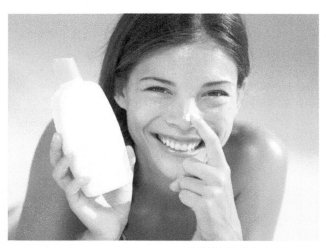

Most sunscreens are formulated to block the sun's rays and prevent making vitamin D in our skin

With the impact of solar exposure, which includes ultraviolet B rays, these compounds are transformed to vitamin D. The circulatory system can then pick up this vitamin D and circulate it to the rest of the body. The ability to both allow these rays to penetrate the skin and the conversion process to vitamin D are products of numerous factors. For instance, the amount and intensity of sun that impacts the skin is a product of where people live, how they dress, how much time they spend in the sun, skin pigment, use of UV-blocking agents on the skin, and age. As a rule, the greater the solar intensity, the lighter the pigment of the skin, the less use of UV-blockers, the greater amount of time exposed to sun, the more skin exposed, and the younger the individual lead to greater production of vitamin D in the skin. Because so much variability exists among these factors, estimating how much vitamin D is coming from body synthesis is too difficult. Consequently, the requirements are based upon what various groups of individuals should be consuming to meet their needs for this vitamin with only minimal solar exposure. Currently, the RDA for vitamin D for most people is 600 IU, while those 70 years and older should consider consuming 800 IU. Although vitamin D is naturally found in some fish and their oils, most of it comes from the consumption of milk and other fortified products. Although this is a required fortification in the United States, many countries do not include vitamin D in milk. Irrespective of the source, many individuals here and abroad are not receiving adequate vitamin D.

Calcitriol: The name used to refer to activated vitamin D, after it has been activated by the kidney and liver.

As discussed later, calcium is essential for the optimal formation and maintenance of bones. Activated vitamin D, known as **calcitriol**, is critical to the absorption of calcium by the small intestine and the kidney's retention of calcium. Contemporary research has demonstrated that calcitriol functions in these sites to produce binding proteins that facilitate absorption of calcium by the small intestinal cells and retention of calcium by renal cells. Newer research is also demonstrating that calcitriol uptake by cells may also result in less potential for some cancerous growth, a reduction in auto-immune diseases like Crohn's disease and rheumatoid arthritis, reduced risk of heart disease, as well as improved use of glucose. Further research will determine whether some of these early studies have significance for the general public.

Minerals

Despite our need for numerous minerals, surprisingly few seem to be commonly inadequate in most diets. As you recall, minerals are inorganic components of our diet that are required, like vitamins, in smaller quantities than the energy-yielding macronutrients.

Calcium, as discussed under the section above regarding vitamin D, is critical for bone growth and maintenance. Recent research has also implicated adequate calcium as a significant factor in the maintenance of appropriate blood pressure, blood clotting, nervous transmission, muscle contraction, and as a cofactor for various significant enzymes. As a result, having adequate calcium outside of the bone as well as inside bones is critical. Recent research has also implicated adequate calcium as a significant factor in the prevention of colon cancer, hypertension, and obesity.

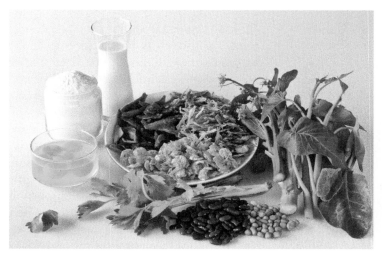

Although dairy products are excellent sources of calcium, other foods also do contain this mineral

To accomplish this balance, the body uses several hormones that either increase the amount of calcium in the bone or increase the amount of calcium in the blood and the rest of the body. More specifically, as discussed previously, one of the most significant hormones is calcitriol, the activated form of vitamin D. As mentioned, this hormone is important in increasing the body's ability to absorb the optimal amount of calcium from food, preventing losses from the urinary tract and balancing calcium levels in bone. Parathyroid hormone is also significant, as it encourages loss of bone with subsequent elevations of blood calcium when needed. If blood calcium starts to rise to levels that are too high, then calcitonin, a hormone secreted by the thyroid gland, will decrease blood calcium.

Calcium is naturally found in milk and other dairy products at higher levels than any other foods, although there are other sources as well. Leafy green vegetables, almonds, and small fish bones are all sources of calcium, but generally have less of this mineral than dairy products and have less capacity for absorption by the human small intestine. Fortunately, the small intestine has mechanisms in place to increase absorption when the levels consumed are low. Many people, feeling either that they cannot get enough calcium from their diet or choose not to do so, have opted to take supplemental calcium. Although research is not yet complete, most

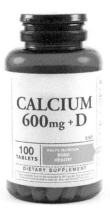

Hydroxyapatite: A substance similar to that found in bone, composed of a matrix of calcium, phosphorus, and hydroxide ion. Typically, in the human body, there are numerous substitutions for these components, including fluoride and magnesium.

Collagen: A protein found in bone, joints, skin, and other areas in the body that provides flexibility to these areas due to the nature of the structure of this protein.

Glycoproteins: Various proteins in the body that also contain sugar components. Some are very significant in ensuring that the other components of our bone, like hydroxyapatite and collagen, are held together properly.

clinicians generally recommend some specific preparations that will be optimally absorbed. A typical recommendation is to take a calcium citrate supplement like Citracal® at a level of about 800 mg/d.

So why is calcium so important for bone? Calcium is part of the matrix of bone called **hydroxyapatite**. This substance is partially composed of calcium as well as phosphorus, another important element, and often fluoride and magnesium. In addition to hydroxyapatite, bone is also composed of proteins called **collagen** and **glycoproteins**. Together they give bone its ability to bend slightly when needed. The disorder known as **osteoporosis** often occurs from inadequate calcium consumption as well as other factors during the life cycle, especially a lack of estrogen that occurs as women mature.

Recently, the Food and Nutrition Board of the Institute of Medicine was requested to evaluate current requirements for calcium. As a result, the RDA's for calcium were set high enough so that a person with about 30% absorption would have a very high probability of obtaining sufficient calcium. During the later teenage years up until age 18, the recommendation was set at 1300 mg/d, reflecting the great needs for calcium during this period of time. Between ages 19 and 50, the requirement was set at a lower level of 1000 mg/d, and for women over age 50 and men and women over age 70, the requirement was set at 1200 mg/d. The increasing risk of osteoporosis in older individuals necessitated the setting of higher levels for these older age groups.

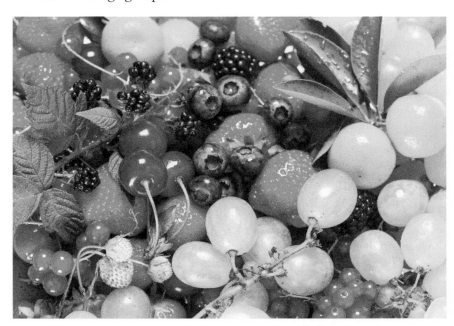

Consuming fresh fruits is an excellent way to get sufficient potassium

Unfortunately, no direct measures are available for determining calcium adequacy, so we have to rely on indirect measures. Right now, the best determinant is to assess dietary intake accurately and be sure it is at least at the standards set by the Food and Nutrition Board. Later in life, perhaps a significant indirect measure is to use equipment such as the **DEXA**, which can determine bone density. The lower bone density is, the more probability that calcium intake has been habitually too low and should be increased.

Potassium is the principal **cation** located inside cells. As such, it is partially responsible for the integrity of cells by maintaining fluid balance with the **intracellular water** surrounding the cells. In addition, potassium plays a critical role in nerve impulse conduction and muscular contractions. In fact, potassium levels are critical for optimal cardiac function.

Although potassium sources are common in various foods, regrettably most Americans do not commonly consume foods such as fresh fruits and vegetables adequately, which could supply us with adequate potassium. Manufacturers of some snack foods, typically high in sodium, have begun to voluntarily add potassium to these foods. Regardless of whether this supplementation is appropriate, it will still result in some increase in potassium intake. The Food and Nutrition Board has recommended an AI of 4700 mg/d of potassium for adults. According to recent surveys, the average American only consumes 3300 mg/d, far below the level suggested. Assessment for potassium status can be accomplished by measuring the levels in plasma.

As a result of inadequate intake or severe fluid losses, potassium deficiency may result in an irregular heart rhythm, muscular weakness, irritability, and disorientation. Recent research also indicates that low body potassium also results in elevated blood pressure and increased probability of death from heart disease. Toxicity from potassium consumption from natural food sources will not occur, but there is some concern that potassium in greatly excessive levels from supplements may cause damage. In fact, injection of high levels of potassium directly into the blood can cause cardiac arrest.

Magnesium is also a major mineral that many Americans often consume inadequately. Although much of our body's magnesium is located in bone, the function there has remained unknown. We do, however, have smaller amounts in our muscles and soft tissues. Magnesium is known to participate in literally hundreds of reactions, primarily those involved in either the extraction or use of energy from protein, fat, or carbohydrate. It would also appear that magnesium is critical to optimal blood pressure regulation and immune system function. Although more research is needed to fully understand its roles in these functions, the consequences of deficiency are clear. Chronic diseases—including heart disease, hypertension, diabetes, and cancer—are all increased by inadequacy of this micronutrient.

Osteoporosis: A disorder occurring more commonly in women of advanced years that involves a reduced amount of bone. Often, osteoporosis leads to bone fractures due to the weakness of the bone.

DEXA: An abbreviation for dual energy x-ray absorptiometry, a technique that can be used to measure bone density or body fat composition.

Cation: A positively charged ion found in the fluids of the body.

Intracellular water: The fluid contained within the various cells of the body.

Anemia

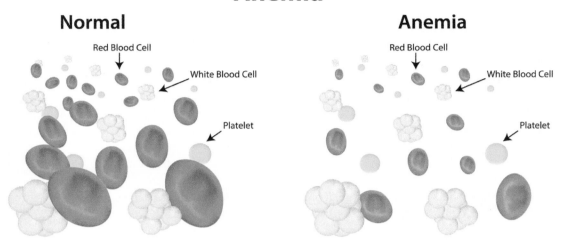

Normal

Red Blood Cell

White Blood Cell

Platelet

Anemia

Red Blood Cell

White Blood Cell

Platelet

Iron deficiency usually results in anemia, with red blood cells decreasing in size from normal

The RDA for magnesium for adult males is 400 mg/d and for women is 310 mg/d. Unfortunately, we do not eat adequate levels because the major sources— including nuts, legumes, whole grains, and green vegetables—are not common foods. Like potassium, toxicity from food is unlikely, but supplements can cause diarrhea and dehydration.

Iron is considered to be a trace element, as the levels found in a 60-kilogram (about 130-pound) man are considerably lower than 30 g and equal about 2.4 g. Despite this low body total, iron is extremely important to optimal body functioning. It has recently been estimated that 1.6 billion people worldwide have iron-deficiency anemia, while in the United States, iron deficiency occurs in approximately 10% of small children as well as female adolescents and those of child-bearing age. Iron is greatly needed during growth, for menstruating females, and for those who are pregnant. It is also not uncommon to find iron-deficiency anemia in older individuals who are losing more blood from their gastrointestinal tract due to aging.

Hematocrit: A measurement of the percentage of packed red blood cells as a part of the total blood volume.

Hemoglobin: A protein produced in the body that uses iron to transport oxygen to tissues and cells that require oxygen.

Fortunately, tremendous work has been accomplished to determine iron status. Although the less specific tests for anemia like the **hematocrit** and **hemoglobin** assays do not pinpoint the source of the anemia, they do provide a screening device so that other tests can be done to more clearly establish iron-deficiency anemia. Consequently, the more sensitive tests for transferrin saturation as well as the serum ferritin assays can be accomplished to determine the source of the anemia as iron deficiency. While the former measures the saturation of an iron transport protein, the latter measures the level of an iron storage protein.

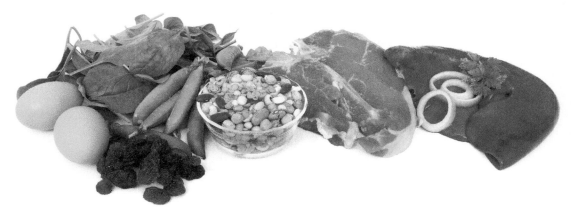

Iron deficiency not only results in the fatigue, weakness, and apathy that accompany anemia but also results in other signs of dysfunction.

For instance, recent research suggests that behavior is affected by iron inadequacy, often before anemia occurs. Primarily due to impaired energy metabolism and alteration of neurotransmitter production, the ability to perform both physical and mental activity is lowered.

Although there are numerous sources of iron available to us, our gastrointestinal tract does not treat all sources as equal. Many of the iron molecules in meat foods are in the **heme** form and are absorbed reasonably well (about 25% of the total), while other molecules in meat foods and all of the iron molecules in plant foods such as legumes and dried fruits are in a **nonheme** form, which is absorbed from just a few percent up to about 17%. As a result, unless an individual in the risk categories cited above consumes large quantities of meat, they are unlikely to have enough iron consumption from food.

Although iron is a required additive to flour products and many people opt to take supplements, the problem of inadequacy persists here and abroad. The RDA for men as well as women over age 50 is 8 mg/d, while women from ages 19 to 50 are recommended to consume 18 mg/d. Levels of intake from supplements and plant foods can be very deceiving with respect to fulfilling the requirements, as the absorption can be considerably lower than the iron from animal foods like red meats, fish, poultry, and eggs.

The focus of this chapter is deficiency, but we also need to be aware of the risk of iron toxicity for some. In addition to acute poisoning often due to toddlers taking iron supplements while not properly supervised, chronic toxicity is also a problem. Iron overload in these small children can result in nausea, vomiting, irregular heartbeat, dizziness, and confusion. Death can be an outcome if help is not sought quickly. As for chronic toxicity, the effects are not as dramatic but are extremely dangerous. It is currently

Although meats are iron-rich foods there are a large variety of non-meat foods with iron

Heme: The type of iron found in foods that is associated with either hemoglobin or similar molecules.

Nonheme: The type of iron found in foods that is not associated with either hemoglobin or similar molecules. It constitutes the majority of iron found in most diets.

believed that iron overload can lead to greater risk of liver failure, some types of cancer, and even heart disease. For these and other reasons, the Food and Nutrition Board has placed a TUL for iron at 45 mg/d.

Suggested Readings

Aigner E, Feldman A, Datz C. Obesity as an emerging risk factor for iron deficiency. *Nutrients.* 2014; 6:3587–3600.

Bendik I, Friedel A, Roos FF, et al. Vitamin D: A critical and essential micronutrient for human health. *Front Physiol.* 2014; 5:248. doi: 10.3389/fphys.2014.00248.

Del Gobbo LC, Imamura F, Wu JH, et al. Circulating and dietary magnesium and risk of cardiovascular disease: A systematic review and meta-analysis of prospective studies. *Am J Clin Nutr.* 2013; 98:160–73.

Fares H, Lavie CJ, DiNicolantonio JJ, O'Keefe JH, Milani RV. Omega-3 fatty acids: A growing ocean of choices. *Curr Atheroscler Rep.* 2014; 16:389. doi: 10.1007/s11883-013-0389-6.

Hunt BD, Cappuccio FP. Potassium intake and stroke risk: A review of the evidence and practical considerations for achieving a minimum target. *Stroke.* 2014; 45:1519–22.

Jones JM. Dietary fiber future directions: Integrating new definitions and findings to inform nutrition research and communication. *Adv Nutr.* 2013; 4:8–15.

Van der Velde RY, Brouwers JR, Geusens PP, Lems WF. Van den Bergh JP. Calcium and vitamin D supplementation: State of the art for daily practice. *Food Nutr Res.* 2014; 58: doi: 10.3402/fnr.v58.21796.

HIGHLIGHT 3

Omega-3 Fatty Acid Intake across the Life Cycle

As discussed within this chapter, consumption of omega-3 fatty acids is of considerable importance. Current research shows that the impact of adequate intake begins in utero and likely continues through the older years. Recent research has shown that the specific fatty acids, EPA and DHA, have shown tremendous benefits for the developing infant. Research on adult subjects has demonstrated benefits of EPA and DHA upon the prevention of cardiovascular disease and some types of cancer, while older adults seem to benefit from EPA and DHA with a reduction in Alzheimer's disease.

Although current dietary guidelines encourage seafood consumption for pregnant women in order to elevate their levels of omega-3 fatty acids, evaluations of maternal intake have demonstrated that the levels of intake are not adequate. With this in mind, investigators have given supplements of EPA or DHA, the most significant omega-3 fatty acids, to pregnant women in order to increase the placental transfer of these fatty acids to the developing fetus. Several promising studies have demonstrated that supplementation to pregnant women has resulted in improved development of their offspring, including problem-solving skills, hand-eye coordination, and a reduction in food allergies. There have also been improvements in pregnancy outcome, such as optimal pregnancy length as opposed to premature delivery.

Male and female adults may also have better protection against cardiovascular disease with optimal intake of omega-3 fatty acids. Numerous studies show that protection against a cardiovascular incident is reduced by the anti-inflammatory effects of EPA or DHA. Even peripheral artery disease, the buildup of plaque in the arteries of the leg, appears to be reduced by appropriate intake of omega-3 fatty acids. The most common type of arrhythmia (irregular beating of the heart) known as atrial fibrillation, often leading to stroke, also seems to be reduced by optimal intake of EPA-DHA.

Recent research in cancer prevention has resulted in several significant correlations between EPA-DHA intake and cancer development. Specifically, high negative correlations seem to exist between intake of omega-3 fatty acids and both breast and prostate cancer. A high negative correlation suggests that higher intakes of these fatty acids reduce the risk of breast and prostate cancer. Although the mechanisms still need exploration, preliminary work suggests that the anti-inflammatory properties of the omega-3 fatty acids are involved in protective mechanisms against these cancers. Other researchers have found that supplementing patients who have undergone cancer therapy will recover faster than those not receiving supplements.

Some studies have shown that individuals with Alzheimer's disease may often have low EPA and DHA blood levels and consequently may experience some degree of improvement with supplementation. At least one study has demonstrated that Alzheimer's patients with only very mild symptoms experienced improvement in cognition with supplementation. Another observed benefit for those with Alzheimer's disease is an improvement in weight gain, which is typically a problem. DHA's presence in neurons and its involvement in the proper functioning of the nervous system provide strong optimism for those researchers and clinicians working to reduce the cognitive impairment caused by Alzheimer's disease.

Suggested Readings

Cederholm T, Salem N Jr, Palmblad J. Omega-3 fatty acids in the prevention of cognitive decline in humans. *Adv Nutr.* 2013; 4:672–6.

Kar S. Role of omega-3 fatty acids in the prevention of atrial fibrillation. *Rev Cardiovasc Med.* 2013; 14:e82–e91.

Lee J.-H. Polyunsaturated fatty acids in children. *PGHN.* 2013; 16:153–61.

Zhang P, Lavoie PM, Lacaze-Masmonteil, et al. Omega-3 long chain polyunsaturated fatty acids for extremely preterm infants: a systematic review. *Pediatrics.* 2014; 134:120–34.

Required Nutrients Found Inadequate Due to Atypical Diets or Lifestyles

Energy-Yielding Macronutrients

Total Carbohydrates

Hydrolyzed: The action where parts of energy-yielding molecules are separated from other components with a resultant release of energy, which is typically how disaccharides and starches are broken down to monosaccharides.

Monosaccharides: Simple sugars that may either be available directly from foods or result from the breakdown of disaccharides or starches. The three major ones are glucose, fructose, and galactose.

Disaccharides: Simple sugars that are a combination of two monosaccharides. The most common ones found in food are sucrose, maltose, and lactose. In the human and animal body, the only one produced is lactose.

In an effort to avoid carbohydrates in their diet, some individuals may inadvertently reduce their total fiber intake as well as their intake of starches and sugars from natural sources. This phenomenon has become increasingly more common as various weight-loss diets encourage less consumption of carbohydrates and greater consumption of protein. As discussed in the previous chapter, both fermentable and nonfermentable fibers are important to health. In addition, maintaining adequate intakes of both natural sources of starch and sugars is essential for health. To understand this phenomena, we must first discuss the role of these carbohydrates in maintaining blood glucose and tissue glycogen. Glucose, a 6-carbon sugar, is the final result of the breakdown of dietary starch, as well as the dietary disaccharides—maltose, sucrose, and lactose. The structure of glucose is shown in Figure 4.1. In the digestive tract, all of these carbohydrates are **hydrolyzed** to **monosaccharides**. You can see from the illustration (Figure 4.2), dietary starch is either composed of branched chains of glucose (amylopectin) or a straight chain of glucose molecules (amylose). The three **disaccharides** are composed of glucose plus glucose (maltose), glucose plus fructose (sucrose), and glucose and galactose (lactose). The monosaccharides, fructose and galactose, are transformed to glucose in the liver; therefore, the commonly consumed disaccharides cited all eventually are transformed to glucose, which enters the blood along with the glucose from starch.

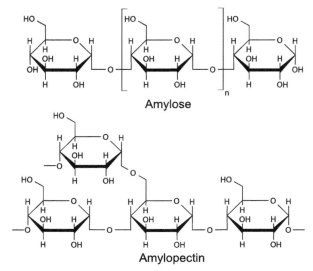

Amylose

Amylopectin

Fig. 4-2: Structure of starches

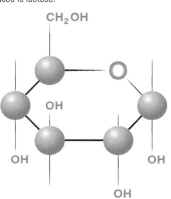

Fig. 4-1: Structure of glucose (note that the blue circles represent carbon atoms)

Glucose Homeostasis

Our bodies rely upon careful regulation of blood glucose, as glucose is an important energy source for many tissues. In particular our **red blood cells** and the cells of the nervous system exclusively rely on glucose as an energy source. Although several hormones, including **insulin** and **glucagon,** are able to control blood glucose so that it is neither too high nor too low, we need to have adequate glucose in our diet so that these hormones can ensure that organs, tissues, and cells can receive the glucose that they need. Although most glucose is stored in our liver as glycogen (see Figure 4.3), a small amount is circulated in our blood. Without adequate levels of carbohydrate intake we deplete our glycogen stores and risk being unable to maintain our blood glucose levels. This problem becomes even more apparent when we engage in endurance activities like running, swimming, and so on. Studies have demonstrated that individuals who consume higher levels of carbohydrate in their diet are able to endure strenuous activity for a longer time than those consuming lower levels of carbohydrate.

Red blood cells: Also known as erythrocytes, these cells carry hemoglobin, which results in their red color. They are critical as an oxygen delivery system to the body's cells.

Insulin: A hormone released by the pancreas that is extremely important in the proper uptake of glucose by many of the body's cells.

Glucagon: A hormone released by the pancreas that results in the release of glucose from body stores of glycogen.

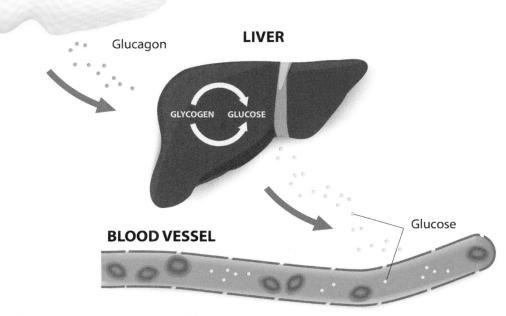

PANCREAS

Glucagon

LIVER

GLYCOGEN   GLUCOSE

Glucose

BLOOD VESSEL

Fig. 4-3: : The pancreas releases glucagon when blood glucose levels fall too low. Glucagon causes the liver to convert stored glycogen into glucose, which is released into the bloodstream.

Protein

When we discuss the special dietary needs of vegetarians in the Highlight section following this chapter, we only briefly describe the problem of inadequate protein intake faced by this population. In addition to vegetarians, some people in this country and a great number of individuals in developing countries do not have access to adequate protein in their diets. Currently the recommended range of protein as a percentage of dietary energy is 10% to 35%. Consuming high amounts of protein still provides energy to the body, and although we think of fat and carbohydrates as key contributors to excess energy intake, protein can be a problem as well. We discuss this issue later in Highlight 7.

Vegetarians

Enzymes: Specific proteins that are involved in either the breakdown, synthesis, or other types of transformation of a variety of molecules in our body.

Although this term describes a very broad group of individuals with different habits, the vegetarians we are concerned about are those who refrain from consumption of all animal products. Because there are about twenty different amino acids in proteins, nine of which are dietarily essential for adults, we need to be sure that we consume these nine amino acids at levels that will provide us with enough of each to form the numerous proteins that we need in our bodies as **enzymes**, hormones, structural components, and other essential materials. In addition, although we are able to produce the eleven nondietarily essential amino acids in our bodies, we typically need to consume many of these so that they can be used for protein production or transformed to other nondietarily essential amino acids through a variety of reactions. Unfortunately, most nonanimal foods are low in some of the essential amino acids, and the protein-producing mechanisms in the body are therefore unable to correctly or adequately produce all of the proteins that are needed. Only a few plant foods, including soy and quinoa, have adequate levels of all of the essential amino acids.

A quinoa salad is a delightful way to consume high quality protein for a vegetarian

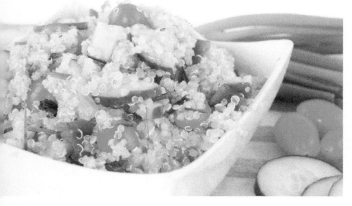

Protein-Deficient Diets

Unfortunately, due to a variety of reasons including poverty, poor food transport systems, or cultural values, many individuals do not consume enough protein nor the essential amino acids that are part of protein. In the United States and other developed countries, poverty often results in food choices that favor caloric intake over nutritional content. One of those nutrients that is typically associated with more expensive food choices is protein. It is not unusual to find people in these developed countries consuming more than adequate calories, resulting in overweight or obesity, yet being nutritionally deficient. In developing countries, any of the reasons cited above—poverty, food transport systems, or cultural values—may contribute to low protein intake. These disorders are so prevalent that they have been given names like **kwashiorkor** and **marasmus**, although as defined, they often result in different types of physiological deficits.

Micronutrients

Vitamin B$_{12}$

Vitamin B$_{12}$ is also commonly found inadequate in the diets of vegans due to their generally refraining from animal foods. There may be some contamination from the microbes that are consumed as part of yogurt or root crops, but research seems to demonstrate that the **bioavailability** of this vitamin from foods other than animal foods is very low. Vitamin B$_{12}$ is important in the appropriate use of folate or folic acid and as a result of deficiency will usually mimic the impact of folic acid deficiency with a form of anemia, referred to as **megaloblastic**, **macrocytic** anemia. This effect is due to the very significant impact that a particular coenzyme derivative of vitamin B$_{12}$ has on the activation of folic acid. This anemia is often referred to as *pernicious anemia*, because it also results in other problems due to the vitamin's involvement in the appropriate use of certain types of fat. If these fats are not metabolized appropriately, then the consequences often are associated with nervous system dysfunction.

Comparison of the red blood cells in macrocytic anemia with normal, microcytic and hypochromic red blood cells.

Kwashiorkor: A nutritional disorder resulting from inadequate protein and calories and that causes edema, fatty liver, and other degenerative changes. It mostly occurs in young children.

Marasmus: A nutritional disorder that results from inadequate protein and calories and causes poor growth and emaciation in children.

Bioavailability: When referring to nutrients, the capacity of the gastrointestinal system to obtain a particular nutrient from food or pharmaceutical sources.

Megaloblastic: A cell that is typified by having an irregular structure. This term commonly refers to red blood cells that are not shaped in their typical ovular form.

Macrocytic: A cell that is smaller than comparable cells of that particular type. This term commonly refers to red blood cells that are smaller than typical red blood cells.

Anemia

| Normal | Microcytic | Macrocytic | Hypochromic |

Vitamin K

To some extent, we depend upon our intestinal microbes to synthesize vitamin K. Vitamin K is essential for the appropriate clotting of both internal and external wounds. If we use antibiotics for a prolonged period, perhaps to diminish an infection of our respiratory system, urinary tract, or some other area, then we also reduce the population of bacteria in our gut, which may be very helpful in providing vitamin K. Most people do not consume the major food sources of vitamin K, like green leafy vegetables, so antibiotic therapy can result in an increased probability of wounds failing to clot in a timely manner.

Water

Most people consume adequate water either through beverage consumption or foods with a high water content, like fruits and vegetables. The human body has several mechanisms in place to be sure that water is maintained at adequate levels, but they have their limits. In the absence of water consumption, dehydration occurs, with serious consequences ranging from initial disorientation to ultimately fatality. The body has two basic ways to try and maintain adequate fluid: thirst sensations and body water conservation. If water is available, then the thirst sensations that come from the tongue or hypothalamus (a part of the brain) will provoke us to consume water or fluid-containing foods. If no or limited water is available, then our body will conserve the water it has through a series of mechanisms beginning with sensing lower water in the blood and ultimately resulting in the kidney reducing losses of fluid in the urine. Although we have some obligatory water losses—such as perspiration, breath moisture, and fecal moisture—in the case of the latter the body reduces the amount of moisture lost in the feces.

Why is water so important? Water is a significant component of our total body mass, usually about 60% of our body mass during our adult years. In fact, infants are born with a considerably greater percentage of water in their bodies, and gradually these high levels are reduced to the 60% cited above. The water in our bodies is important in many ways. Perhaps the most significant is the transport of materials throughout the body. Our cardiovascular system is the major linkage between the organs of our body. The heart, the center of this system, pumps the materials in our arterio-venous system from points of intake like our lungs and small intestine as well as from secretory organs like our liver and the various **endocrine** organs throughout our bodies. Another very significant impact that water has in our bodies is as a medium for the occurrence of biochemical reactions and the deposition of electrolytes. Electrolytes, including potassium, chloride, and sodium, have significant roles in nervous conduction and muscle movement. Another very significant role of body water is structural. As mentioned earlier, over half of our bodies are composed of water. This lends structure to the bones, muscles, fat, and organs that are all important components of our body. Water can also be a significant provider of protection for our bodies in several ways. Along with fat, it provides cushioning for the organs in our body in the event of contact with a hard surface. Second, it provides our bodies with a cooling mechanism; when we sweat, we are able to cool off and prevent overheating. Recent research also suggests that water intake can affect mood.

Endocrine: A term that refers to the organs of the system responsible for the release of hormones in the body.

Suggested Readings

Hunt A, Harrington D, Robinson S. Vitamin B$_{12}$ deficiency. *BMJ*. 2014; 349: g5226.

Pross N, Demazieres A, Girard N, et al. Effects of changes in water intake on mood of high and low drinkers. *PLoS One*. 2014; 9:e94754.

Rodriguez NR, DiMarco NM, Langley S. Position of the American Dietetic Association, Dietitians of Canada, and the American College of Sports Medicine: Nutrition and athletic performance. 2009; 109:509–27.

Shearer MJ, Fu X, Booth SL. Vitamin K nutrition, metabolism, and requirements: Current concepts and future research. *Adv Nutr*. 2012; 3:182–95.

Westerterp-Plantenga MS, Lemmens SG, Westerterp KR. Dietary protein—its role in satiety, energetics, weight loss, and health. *Br J Nutr*. 2012; 108 Supplement 2:S105–S112.

HIGHLIGHT 4

Special Nutritional Needs of Vegetarians

Several of the nutrients discussed in this chapter are often consumed inadequately by vegetarians. The common meaning of this term has traditionally been used to describe a person who does not eat animal meat. More recently, due to variability in dietary preferences, new terms like vegans have emerged to describe those who not only refrain from animal meats but also do not consume the products of animals, such as milk and eggs. There is also a wide range of individuals between these two types. Some vegetarians eat the flesh of seafood but not other animals. We refer to them as pisco-vegetarians. If this sounds confusing, then the rationale for some of these behaviors is even more bewildering. Reasons for these behaviors include environmental, health, and spiritual concerns as well as the taste and texture of various foods. Most humans are omnivores, meaning that they consume plant and animal foods. Interestingly some people are carnivores, eating only animal foods. A study of these behaviors is beyond the scope of this highlight and has been reviewed extensively by many others, but it will not provide us with an understanding of the special nutritional needs that vegetarians face.

A large body of evidence also links various forms of vegetarianism to more optimal health. In particular, research observations have linked the reduced or complete elimination of animal meats and products to reductions in heart disease, diabetes mellitus, obesity and specific types of cancer, such as colon cancer. This effect has also been reviewed extensively by many others in the field of nutrition and disease, but does not provide us with insight into the special nutritional needs of vegetarians.

Several of the most difficult nutrients to consume in a vegetarian diet have been discussed in this chapter as well as the previous chapter. These include vitamin B_{12}, protein, omega-3 fatty acids, vitamin D, and calcium. Let's begin with those nutrients covered in this chapter and then discuss the other nutrients afterward.

Vitamin B_{12}

Vitamin B_{12} is virtually absent in plant materials, and even though there may be some contaminating microbes on root crops like carrots and turnips, as well as tempeh, algae, and sea vegetables, the materials made by these microbes are either poorly bioavailable or not made in a form that is useful to humans. Consequently, the vegan has little chance of satisfying the requirement for vitamin B_{12} through nonfortified dietary sources. Vegans generally are dependent upon a supplement of some sort, either a multivitamin or fortified foods with B_{12} like soy or breakfast cereals. The vegetarian who does not eat meat but still consumes fish, eggs, or milk will likely not be at risk for deficiency.

Protein and Amino Acids

As discussed earlier in this chapter, we need to consume not just adequate amounts of protein but also adequate levels of essential amino acids to ensure that we produce the appropriate proteins our bodies need. With the exception of soy and quinoa, plant products do not have the correct levels of essential amino acids. Vegans who consume soy or quinoa are likely not at risk, but people who adhere to a nonanimal food diet and do not consume soy or quinoa regularly need to complement their plant food consumption. Complementation means eating a combination of plant foods where one is low in a particular essential amino acid but adequate in the others while the other one is low in a different essential amino acid but adequate in the others. A good example is complementing grains with legumes, where the former is generally low in lysine, tryptophan, and threonine and the latter low in methionine. As before, we are not very concerned about the vegetarian who eats fish, milk, or eggs, since all of these are generally adequate in all of the essential amino acids.

Omega-3 Fatty Acids

The importance of consuming this type of polyunsaturated fat at adequate levels was discussed in the previous chapter. Although there are omega-3 fatty acids in terrestrial foods such as flax and flaxseed, canola, and olive oil, the transformation to the types of omega-3 fatty acids known to be important to health is low. Vegans, due to not eating any animal foods, will be at a loss to acquire EPA and DHA from their diet, and vegetarians who do not consume marine animals. This lack of EPA and DHA in nonmarine foods has led to both fortification of foods and supplementation with capsules and oils. Research has led to the fortification of eggs through the supplementation of laying chickens as well as the addition of EPA and DHA to products like margarine. Others rely upon either gel capsules containing fish oils or the fish oils taken in liquid form. Recently, capsules have been produced which contain extracts of marine algae, which are believed to provide adequate amounts of omega-3 fatty acids. This would provide a non-animal food

alternative for the vegan, but further studies need to be done on the bioavailability from these capsules.

Vitamin D

As discussed in chapter 3, many people do not obtain enough vitamin D in their diet to maintain optimum health. Although some of the same reasons apply to vegetarians due to a very limited choice of foods that have vitamin D, those who consume neither fish nor dairy are particularly prone to low vitamin D intake. As with omega-3 fatty acids, choices include the consumption of fortified foods like margarines and breakfast cereals or vitamin D supplements. Unlike omega-3 fatty acids, a third choice is to attempt to expose one's skin to enough sunlight to result in transformation of a cholesterol-like substance in skin to vitamin D. There are several obstacles to this strategy, however, including the lack of strong sunlight in areas distant from the equator, reduced transformation due to dark skin pigment or aging, and the contemporary use of sun-blocking agents, which not only prevent skin cancer but also prevent sunlight from transforming the precursors in skin to vitamin D.

Calcium intake has been a problem for many people, as discussed in the previous chapter. The vegetarian who opts not to consume dairy products, however, is particularly at risk of inadequacy. Alternative sources among plant materials includes almonds and some leafy green vegetables. Fish with edible bones like sardines or canned salmon with bones that can be ground up in a food processor and made into patties are an alternative for the pisco-vegetarian. Many vegetarians opt for the fortified products available, including juices such as orange juice, milk substitutes like soy and almond milk, mineral water, or the myriad of breakfast cereals with added calcium. Others turn to supplements such as the common calcium carbonate tablet or the more absorbable calcium citrate tablet.

Suggested Readings

Craig WJ. Nutrition concerns and health effects of vegetarian diets. *Nutr Clin Pract.* 2010; 25:613–20.

Lane K, Derbyshire E, Li W, et al. Bioavailability and potential uses of vegetarian sources of omega-3 fatty acids: A review of the literature. *Crit Rev Food Sci Nutr.* 2014; 54:572–9.

McEvoy CT, Temple N, Woodside JV. Vegetarian diets, low-meat diets and health: A review. *Public Health Nutrition.* 2012; 15:2287–94.

Ruby MB. Vegetarianism: A blossoming field of study. *Appetite.* 2012; 58:141–50.

Watanabe F, Yabuta Y, Tanioka Y et al. Biologically active vitamin B_{12} compounds in foods for preventing deficiency among vegetarian and elderly subjects. *J Agric Food Chem.* 2013; 61:6769–75.

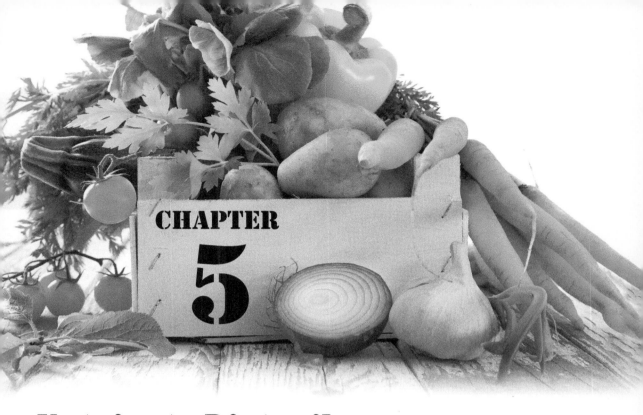

Nutrients Dietarily Adequate Due to Fortification of Foods

The FDA (U.S. Food and Drug Administration) has required the food industry to add nutrients to various foods since the 1920s. The industry complies with these laws and sometimes voluntarily adds nutrients back to their foods that have been inadvertently removed during processing, or enriches foods with nutrients that are not normally found in these foods. As we understand more about the needs for various nutrients, the FDA and the food industry both respond with the addition of various nutrients. In this chapter I focus on the major nutrients that are added to food, which otherwise would likely be inadequate in the diets of most Americans if those nutrients were not added.

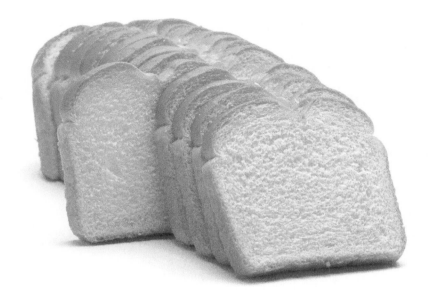

In the US, the FDA has mandated that flour be enriched, so that even highly milled grains used for white bread still have an abundance of added nutrients

In previous chapters we discussed several of these added nutrients, which, despite either FDA requirements or voluntary addition by the industry, still persist as being inadequate in the U.S. diet for many individuals. As discussed in chapter 3, this included omega-3 fatty acids, calcium, vitamin D, and iron. The first two of these have been added to various foods voluntarily by the food industry, while vitamin D has been added to milk and iron is a nutrient that has been added to grain products due to FDA requirements. Several other nutrients have also been added to grain products due to FDA requirements, including thiamin, riboflavin, niacin, and folic acid. These are all discussed in this chapter, as they have had a very significant impact upon the U.S. dietary consumption of these nutrients. In addition, the FDA has virtually eradicated both iodine and fluoride deficiency in the United States due to its compulsory addition of these nutrients to commonly consumed foods and beverages.

Thiamin

The need for thiamin to prevent deficiency symptoms has been known for about 200 years. Despite this knowledge, thiamin deficiency is still present throughout the world. The Food and Drug Administration, however, deemed it necessary that grain products manufactured in the United States should have reasonable levels of thiamin in order to prevent these deficiencies. Globally, we still see several types of thiamin deficiency. The deficiency disorders are known as *wet beriberi* and *dry beriberi*. The former is characterized by muscle weakness and wasting, while the latter is mostly

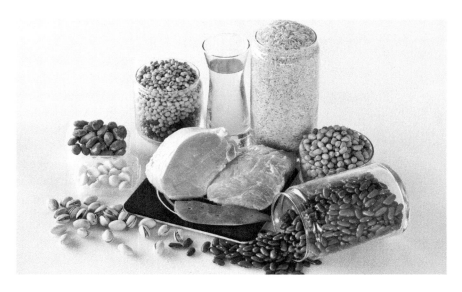

Foods contributing to thiamin intake

characterized by a rapidly beating and enlarged heart. The appearances are very different, with wet beriberi resulting in **edema** and dry beriberi usually resulting in an emaciated look. Currently in the United States, the only risk groups for deficiency are alcoholics, the elderly, and some people taking **diuretics** for health reasons, resulting in serious losses of the vitamin. Although the health value was discovered in the late nineteenth century, not until the 1930s was the structure determined. Due to its high content in enriched and whole grains as well in other foods like pork, beef, salmon, and legumes, there is adequate thiamin in most diets, as mentioned earlier. The RDA for adult males is set at 1.2 mg/d, and for adult females, 1.1 mg/d. In order to be physiologically active, two phosphate groups are added to its structure, producing thiamin diphosphate. This coenzyme is active in many reactions, which result in the production of energy as adenosine triphosphate (ATP) and responsible for materials used in nucleic acid and fat synthesis. There is little evidence for toxic effects due to thiamin intake, and consequently there is no UL established for it.

Edema: Accumulation of fluid in the interstitial space, the area between our cells, and our vascular system. Usually results in a bloated appearance.

Diuretics: Medicines that encourage loss of body fluid; often used to reduce edema.

Riboflavin

Riboflavin is also not currently a problem in the U.S. diet. Deficiency is not known in the United States, and even those individuals in other places in the world with riboflavin deficiency only experience distress without life-threatening illness. Typically after several months of poor intake, individuals experience skin and oral lesions. Discovery of the vitamin occurred around the same time as thiamin, with the structure determined also in the 1930s. Because of the

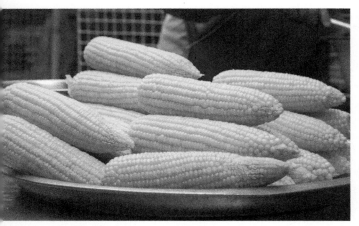

Corn is a delicious food filled with many nutrients, but not tryptophan nor niacin.

fortification of flour and riboflavin's high presence in breakfast cereals as well as numerous other foods, we do not need to be concerned with our intake when consuming a typical diet. The RDA for adults is set at 1.3 mg/d for males and 1.1 mg/d for females. The vitamin is transformed to either of two coenzymes, flavin mononucleotide (FMN) and flavin adenine dinucleotide (FAD), both of which are important in enhancing various metabolic reactions, including the extraction of energy from fat, carbohydrate, and protein.

Niacin

Although we no longer have a large number of people in the United States with niacin deficiency, this was not the case before the early part of the twentieth century. Due to the efforts of Dr. Joseph Goldberger, who investigated the crisis of pellagra in the southern United States, he found that the disease was due to lack of niacin primarily due to the poorer classes' reliance upon corn products. Although pellagra had been known in Europe for centuries, it was always thought to be a vector-borne disease, like the plague. Goldberger's observations that only the inmates in mental institutions had pellagra—but not the caretakers—led to this remarkable discovery.

Niacin deficiency can result in fatality due to its effects upon the gastrointestinal tract, resulting in diarrhea, vomiting, and nausea. In addition, other effects result in severe dermatitis, primarily in response to solar exposure to the skin, as well as dementia with memory loss and confusion.

The requirements for niacin are somewhat complicated because, in addition to dietary sources of niacin, our bodies can transform excess tryptophan (an amino acid) to niacin. Consequently we use the term *niacin equivalents* when discussing recommendations for niacin. The RDA for adults is 16 mg NE/d for men and 14 mg NE/d for women. It is presumed that in the United States about half of our intake comes from tryptophan conversion and the other half from fortified cereals and grains as well as natural sources of various meats and fish. Niacin functions as part of the structure of nicotinamide adenine dinucleotide (NAD) and nicotinamide adenine dinucleotide phosphate (NADP). While the former is primarily involved in energy production from carbohydrate, protein, and fat, the latter is used to enhance the production of fat and DNA (deoxyribonucleic acid), the basis of our genetic structures. Unlike with thiamin and riboflavin, the Food and Nutrition Board is concerned about possible toxic effects including flushing and headaches, so a UL for supplements and fortified foods has been set at 35 mg/d. A very high dose of nicotinic acid, a derivative of niacin, is sometimes used to reduce low-density lipoprotein (LDL). This carrier of cholesterol travels in the blood and deposits cholesterol in tissues, including our arteries, which can result in enhancement of cardiovascular disease. The typical dose level is 6 g/d, far higher than would be consumed on a typical diet. Recent evidence, however, has disputed the claim that nicotinic acid is helpful. Further research needs to be accomplished to determine whether nicotinic acid does indeed reduce LDL.

Folic Acid

Although there is still some evidence of lower than adequate folic acid or folate (as it is often called) intake in the United States, the 1998 FDA mandate to require folic acid fortification of flour products has been very successful in reducing the level of inadequacy as well as the consequences. Let's first discuss the problem of inadequate body folic acid. Individuals may experience inadequacy for many reasons in addition to low intake, including inadequate body levels of vitamin B_{12} as discussed in Chapter 4, malabsorption, and use of prescription drugs that interfere with folic acid use. An example of such a drug is methotrexate, long used for its ability to fight certain cancers as well as rheumatoid arthritis.

The history of folic acid discovery goes back to the 1870s, when liver was fed to patients with a specific type of anemia. This anemia is known as *megaloblastic macrocytic anemia*, described in the previous chapter as typified by the presence of large, irregularly shaped red blood cells. As with many of the vitamins, the structure was not established until several decades into the twentieth century, primarily due to obstacles in research techniques and equipment. Although the presence of anemia is certainly a major deficiency sign, others include fatigue, headaches, shortness of breath,

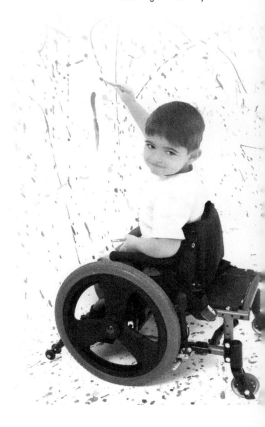

Folic acid deficiency can result in neurological damage during gestation resulting in disability

and a rapid heartbeat. Although not affecting the general population, a major thrust of the FDA mandate was to try to eradicate the neurological problems that often result in infants born to folate-deficient mothers.

As with niacin, the requirement has become complicated and we currently use μg DFE (dietary folate equivalents) to incorporate both natural dietary intake of folic acid as well as fortified or supplemented folic acid found in flour and other foods and supplements as well. A large part of the complication in determining requirements is the fact that supplements have a higher bioavailability than natural sources of folate. A major reason is the more absorbable structure of synthetic folate as opposed to the natural structure, which requires enzymatic alteration. Although the RDA for both male and nonpregnant female adults is 400 μg DFE/d, 1 μg of natural food folate is equal to 1 μg DFE, while between 0.5 and 0.6 μg of supplemental folate is equal to 1 μg DFE. The requirement for pregnant women is 600 μg DFE due to the large amount needed for proper neurological development of the fetus. According to the most recent NHANES results, 85% of the U.S. population was receiving adequate folic acid.

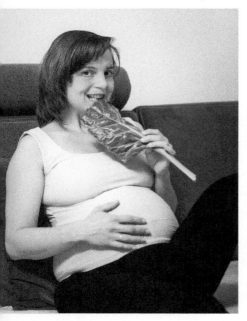

Aside from the fortified products like grains, flour, cereals, and orange juice, natural sources include green vegetables, legumes, and fruits, although raw foods have a higher level since most cooking and processing techniques either destroy or otherwise remove folate from foods.

There are at least four coenzymatic derivatives of folic acid, each with specific functions, but primarily the purpose is to transfer single-carbon functional groups to metabolites that require them for their function. Some of the more significant functions include nucleic acid and methionine synthesis. A variety of tests are used to determine folic acid status, including measurement of folic acid in various fragments of the blood as well as urinary excretion. About 11 to 28 mg of folic acid are stored in the body, with about half in the liver. There have been reports of folic acid toxicity, with 15 mg of food folate associated with insomnia, tiredness, irritability, and gastrointestinal effects. More serious concerns have been raised for synthetic folate, with the UL set at 1 mg due to an increase in neurological issues and possibly an increase in some types of cancer.

Green leafy vegetables are a great source of folic acid

Despite these concerns, numerous health benefits have been associated with adequate intake of folate, including prevention of cardiovascular disease and stroke, Alzheimer's disease, and cancer of the lung and the gastrointestinal tract. As mentioned earlier, the prevention of neural tube defects, such as spina bifida, in infants by encouraging closure of the verte-bra has resulted in significantly less incidence of this disorder. The current evidence suggests that the primary disorder is genetic in nature, but that adequate levels of folic acid can override the genetic predisposition.

Iodine

Despite a current absence of iodine deficiency in the United States, global deficiency persists as a very serious sit-uation. In fact, it is the most prevalent nutritional deficiency worldwide, with 300 million individuals suffering from its effects. In adults who become iodine inadequate, the primary effect is goiter, an enlargement of the thyroid gland. This secretory gland, located in the neck, is responsible for the secretion of an iodine-containing hormone to many tissues of the body. Most adults

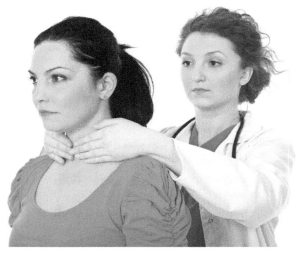

with low iodine intake manage to still get enough iodine to produce these hormones, because goiter involves an enlargement of the thyroid in order to pick up as much iodine as possible coming from the diet. Other than enlargement of the thyroid gland, generally no physiological or metabolic changes take place in the adult with low iodine intake.

A simple check of the size of the thyroid in the neck will detect goiter

Unfortunately for children, the consequences of low dietary iodine are much more serious. The iodine deficiency disorders (IDDs) general-ly result in profound metabolic and physiologic changes in an infant or child. Perhaps the most obvious result is a failure to grow, resulting from the disorder called "cretinism." Cretinism also results in other changes that are detrimental to the growing child, including neurological issues such as mental deficiency, deafness, and a lack of appropriate motor skills. Not so obvious, iodine deficiency in children can also result in thyroid organ failure. The thyroid is involved in general development as well as regulation of metabolic activity, resulting in even more serious problems for children.

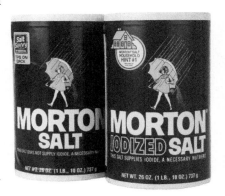

Fortunately, appropriate dietary levels of iodine can correct cretinism in infants and children. Since 1924 the FDA mandated the selling of iodized salt, which in-cludes potassium iodide. The consumer has the option of

purchasing the iodized salt or salt without iodine. Relying upon the food industry to use iodized salt in their products would be impractical, as they do not need to do so nor indicate whether iodized salt is in their products. We do receive some unintended iodine in manufactured food products like bread due to an iodine-containing preservative used, as well as the iodine in milk and other dairy products resulting from milking machines that are cleaned with an iodine-containing antibacterial compound. The iodine in salt becomes increasingly important to individuals living in mountainous or lowland noncoastal areas, as the plants and animals in these areas receive little iodine from the soil. For those living near the coasts, aquatic plants like kelp and marine fish like cod represent reliable sources of iodine. For adults, the RDA is 150 µg/d while due to the high needs of the fetus and newborn, the RDA for pregnant women is 220 µg/d while the RDA for breast-feeding women is 290 µg/d! Various blood, urine, and ultrasound tests can be used for determining iodine deficiency and goiter.

As mentioned earlier, iodine is taken up solely by the thyroid gland for the production of hormones. These hormones interact with our cells and organs to result in increased oxygen consumption and heat generation, primarily through increased **basal metabolic rate (BMR)**. In the neonate, these hormones also encourage neurological development and overall growth.

Fortunately, we absorb iodine very well in our small intestine, about 90% of what we typically consume. Quite obviously, most of our bodily iodine is stored in our thyroid gland. Toxicity is uncommon, but there is a UL of 1.1 mg/d, as some have experienced nausea, vomiting, diarrhea, and fever from high intakes.

Basal metabolic rate (BMR): The rate at which an individual uses energy irrespective of activity and other factors. It is usually dependent mostly on fat-free mass, gender, and age.

Adequate fluoride intake leads to prevention of tooth decay.

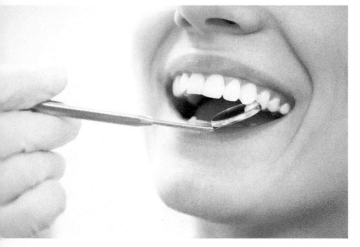

Fluoride

Although it is difficult to consider water a food, it is certainly an essential nutrient. As discussed in chapter 4, the consequences of inadequate fluid in the body are serious and can lead to death. Fluoride has been added to the drinking water of many municipalities since the 1950s and is currently added to most public water supplies at a level that should provide people with a safe and adequate amount. The level used is about 1 mg/l. Initial and subsequent studies demonstrate that children and adolescents not provided with adequate fluoride will be more prone to dental caries (cavities) as a result. The scientific community is still equivocal concerning the role of fluoride in the strength of other bones. As a result of some of this uncertainty, the Food and Nutrition Board has determined that fluoride requirements should be expressed as adequate intakes (AIs). The AI for male adults is 4 mg/d, and for female adults, 3 mg/d.

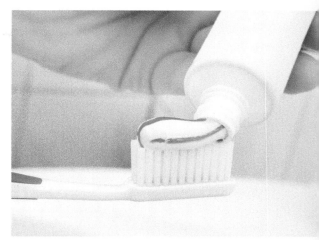

Most children, adolescents, and adults can rely upon the fluoride levels in public drinking water for adequacy. What other sources are available to those who do not have this resource? Fish with bones, legumes, and decaffeinated teas seem to be the most reliable food sources for fluoride. In addition, particularly for infants or young children, fluoride drops can be obtained by prescription and used to add fluoride to water or other beverages.

Adequate fluoride intake leads to prevention of tooth decay.

Why is fluoride so important for the adequate structure of teeth? Fluoride is apparently an essential component of dentin and enamel, the outside shells of teeth. These shells need to resist the destructive effects of acid produced by bacteria that inhabit the mouth—in particular, streptococcus mutans.

Somewhat unusually, we absorb most of our fluoride through our stomachs, as opposed to the small intestine, which is more typical for most nutrients. In fact, we absorb almost all of the fluoride we consume. Out of the fluoride absorbed into the blood, almost all of it goes to our teeth. Injudicious use of fluoride supplements, overconsumption of toothpaste with fluoride, or consumption of drinking water with extremely high levels of fluoride (as is sometimes the case in the southwestern United States) can result in a toxicity to teeth known as *fluorosis*. Fluorosis first appears as chalky white spots on the teeth, followed by brown spots and weakening of the teeth.

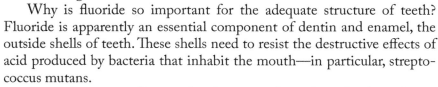

Suggested Readings

Czeizel AE, Dudas I, Vereczkey A, et al. Folate deficiency and folic acid supplementation: The prevention of neural-tube defects and congenital heart defects. *Nutrients*. 2013; 5:4760–75.

Lanska DJ. Historical aspects of the major neurological vitamin deficiency disorders: The water-soluble B vitamins. *Handb Clin Neurol.* 2010; 95:445–76.

Moyer VA. Prevention of dental caries in children from birth through age 5 years: U.S. Preventive Task Force recommendation statement. *Pediatrics.* 2014; 133:1102–11.

Zhou SJ, Anderson AJ, Gibson RA, et al. Effect of iodine supplementation in pregnancy on child development and other clinical outcomes: A systematic review of randomized controlled trials. *Am J Clin Nutr.* 2013; 98: 1241–54.

HIGHLIGHT 5

The Future of "Designer Foods"

Chapter 5 focused upon nutrients that in most cases have been added to food as a result of U.S. government mandates to the food industry to enrich various foods with selected nutrients. In general, the nutrients required represent a response to public health problems throughout the country with respect to the inadequacy of certain nutrients in various target groups. This type of enrichment differs from the industry-based decision to add various nutrients to foodstuffs that will increase the nutritional value of the foods, providing additional ways that individuals can receive the nutrients they require. For instance, the addition of calcium to orange juice creates a new source of calcium for individuals who do not want to take a supplement or cannot or will not consume dairy products. This perspective is not intended to provide an encyclopedic or comprehensive listing of all the ways that the food industry is bringing us designer foods, but rather some examples of current uses and future ways that the food industry can improve our dietary intake.

One interesting area is the introduction of functional fibers to various foods. Functional fibers primarily differ from the fibrous materials naturally found in foodstuffs due either to their being produced in the laboratory or extracted from plant or animal materials and placed in other foods that would not normally have these extracted substances. Functional fiber typically is similar to dietary fiber in that it is nondigestible by human enzymes and there is some evidence that it provides health benefits to humans who consume it. There are numerous examples of functional fiber. Many are extracted from plants and are already found in many of the foods we commonly eat as a fiber source. For instance, cellulose, pectin, lignin, gums, β-glucans, fructans, psyllium, polyols, and resistant starches, although considered to be functional fibers, are already consumed naturally as a component of other foods. Several extracts of the shells of crab, shrimp, and lobster as well as the exoskeletons of insects, chitin, and chitosan may also prove to be valuable functional fibers for humans as more research accumulates to show positive physiological effects. Other potential functional fibers are produced from various materials such as polydextrose and resistant dextrins, which are carbohydrate derivatives. These last two also require evidence of positive physiological effects in humans in order to be included as true functional fibers. Some current uses of the addition of functional fibers are with meat, meatballs, and biscuits. Some of these functional fibers are also prebiotics, carbohydrates that encourage the proliferation of beneficial bacteria in the colon. Cereals and margarine are two good examples of foods that have incorporated prebiotics.

Another example of designer foods are those that include omega-3 fatty acids as an additive. Without question, this type of fatty acid is physiologically significant for health and therefore should be considered a functional fat. As previously mentioned, omega-3's are added to margarine as well as fed to laying chickens to enrich the omega-3 content of their eggs. Current research is also focusing on the micro-encapsulation of fish oils and their introduction to yogurt, bread, cereal products, milk, mayonnaise, salad dressings, and crackers.

Others have taken the approach that various components of meat can be introduced to enrich the nutritional value of foods. Meat hydrolysates have been introduced to condiments, sauces, and soups to improve the protein quality of these products.

A myriad of examples are available of the introduction of vitamins and minerals to various foodstuffs to improve their nutritional value. Perhaps the most common has been additives to breakfast cereals. In addition to the required fortification with thiamin, riboflavin, niacin, folic acid, and iron, many manufacturers also add the minerals calcium and zinc plus vitamins A, B_6, B_{12}, C, D, and E. Another recent example has been the addition of potassium to potato chips.

Most of us are confused when it comes to trying to identify the health values of phytochemicals—plant components that have biological activity in humans, animals, or cellular systems. There are literally thousands of phytochemicals in plants, some of which do appear to have health value. Most of these phytochemicals need to be consumed in large quantities to have a physiological impact. Although many are therefore consumed as capsules or pills, some are used as food additives.

Recent surveys have shown which phytochemicals appear in the greatest amounts in our nutrient intake. Perhaps the most significant conclusion from this research is that individuals who meet the USDA guidelines for fruit and vegetable intake come the closest to consuming these phytochemicals suspected of having physiological value. The categories that are most prevalent in our diet and for which there is some evidence of physiological value are the carotenoids and phenolics.

Among the carotenoids, the greatest amount of research has focused upon α-carotene, β-carotene, lutein, zeaxanthin, β-cryptoxanthin, and lycopene because of their high content in fruits and vegetables and concentration in various human fluids and organs. Among phenolics, most research has focused upon anthocyanins, hesperitin, quercetin, and ellagic acid. Recent research shows the potential for some of these nutrients in disease prevention. For the carotenoids, disease prevention includes heart disease, macular degeneration, and prostate cancer. Phenolics show potential for anticancer activity, anti-inflammatory activity, inhibition of bone loss, and prevention of cognitive and motor function decreases with aging. These phytochemicals are all candidates for addition to designer foods and are appearing primarily in beverages.

Probiotics are finding their way into numerous foodstuffs. They are basically live cultures of bacteria that are intended to colonize the large intestine to improve digestive function.

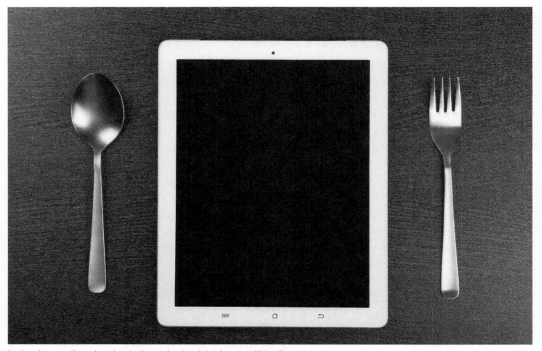

Its hard to predict what the designer foods of the future will be like

Although yogurt has been the main product used to incorporate these bacteria, other dairy products and fruit juices have also been used.

Although taste has been demonstrated to be the main determinant of consumer acceptability of these altered products, sociodemographic factors also seem to predict consumption. Most studies in the United States demonstrate that the typical consumer of these types of products is a female, older than 55, in a higher income class, and well-educated. Purchase and consumption of designer foods appear to provide consumers with a modern and positive impression of themselves and a pathway toward a healthy lifestyle that deviates from the conventional diets advised by nutrition experts. This positive attitude translates into a trend toward increased purchase of these designer foods.

Suggested Readings

Hathwar SC, Rai AK, Modi VK, et al. Characteristics and consumer acceptance of healthier meat and meat product formulations—a review. *J Food Technol.* 2012; 49:653–64.

Ozen AE, Pons A, Tur JA. Worldwide consumption of functional foods: A systematic review. *Nutr Rev.* 2012; 70:472–81.

Siro I, Kapoina E, Kapoina B, et al. Functional food: Product development, marketing and consumer acceptance—a review. *Appetite.* 2008; 51:456–67.

Nutrients Typically Adequate but Not Excessive in Most Diets

Numerous vitamins and minerals are found in most people's diets despite how erratically they might eat. Some are found in high levels as they are needed by the body in large quantities, while others are found at low levels corresponding to the small amounts needed to preserve health. Some of these vitamins and minerals are often found in general supplements or as single sources. Unless an individual has a greater than normal need for these nutrients, it is likely unnecessary to purchase and consume supplements including these nutrients.

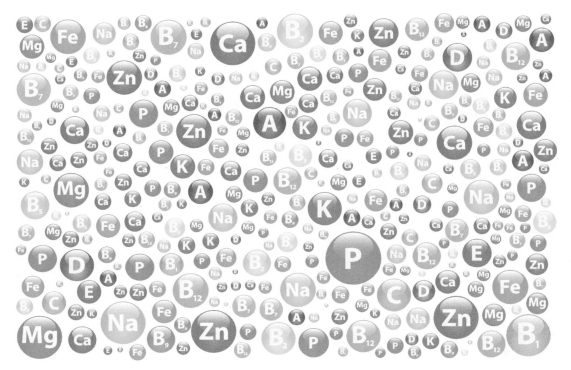

Vitamins

Biotin is rarely found as a deficiency among people. Almost the only way one can become deficient would be to eat a huge amount of raw egg whites with their biotin source. A protein called avidin can bind with the biotin but only when the egg whites have not been cooked, which destroys the natural form of the protein. This is a very unlikely case and has rarely been seen. In the few cases that have been documented, the effects of deficiency have been benign, with skin rash and hair loss. Biotin is used only in very small amounts in the body, and more than enough is in most food groups. Toxicity is also quite unlikely, and no UL is identified with it. Although biotin is not important nutritionally, it does have great significance biochemically in the body, with a very important role in metabolism, particularly fat utilization. There is no transformation of biotin to a more active form, and in its naturally consumed form biotin carries carbon dioxide to be used in metabolism.

Choline has only recently been identified as a vitamin, despite the many years it has been known to be involved in metabolism. Specifically choline is now known to be required in the diet for the formation of acetylcholine, a neurotransmitter, and for phosphatidyl choline, an important component

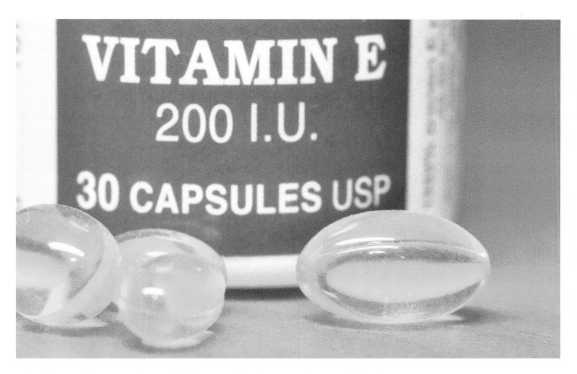

of cell membranes. Overall, these and other products of choline are important for brain development and cognition. In humans, a major deficiency sign is fatty liver and liver dysfunction. In newborns, deficiency cause a greater rate of birth defects, particularly in the form of neural tube disorders. This effect is the same as that which occurs with folic acid inadequacy. Although the American Academy of Pediatrics suggests fortification of infant formulas; however, despite a slightly lower intake by adults than is suggested, there is no current movement to encourage adults to take supplements or to fortify foods. Some evidence exists of toxicity at intake levels over ten times the adequate intake level due to possible hypotension that may occur, but it would be unusual to find these levels in the diet.

Pantothenic acid is not commonly deficient in most diets as it is found in reasonable amounts in most foods. Although it has little nutritional significance, pantothenic acid has great biochemical significance as a component of coenzyme A, which is very important for energy use, synthesis of fat, and neurotransmitter synthesis. At this time, no toxicity has been assigned.

Vitamin E was originally described as any of eight different compounds with similar structure. Recently, all but one of these have been eliminated from food tables as being useful to fulfill the requirement for vitamin E. The one structure is known as alpha-tocopherol and it has the best capacity

Antioxidant: A chemical substance that reduces the capacity of other chemicals to result in oxidation of biological structures or materials.

Free radicals: Chemical substances that typically can attack DNA, RNA, and proteins, often damaging them so that they are no longer useful.

to be transported in the human body, acting as an **antioxidant** to prevent the attack of **free radicals** on cellular membranes. Through the consumption of oils (particularly polyunsaturated ones) as well as nuts, seeds, and wheat germ, we appear to be getting adequate consumption. As I discuss later, we actually consume more gamma-tocopherol than alpha-tocopherol, but this particular tocopherol does not appear to either be transported in the body very well, or to prevent damage to cellular membranes.

Vitamin E deficiency was first discovered in animals in the 1920s and appeared to prevent fetal destruction in pregnant female rats. More recently, deficiency has also been found to result in destruction of muscles in rats, somewhat similar to muscular dystrophy in humans. Neither of these deficiency signs have been demonstrated in humans despite very low intakes of vitamin E; however, some deficiency signs do appear in human subjects. When very low levels of vitamin E are present, a greater rate of destruction of red blood cells appears to occur. This condition is not common and appears to occur only rarely in response to disorders of fat malabsorption like cystic fibrosis.

Contemporary research suggests that alpha-tocopherol may also enhance our immune response as well as prevent heart disease and some types of cancer; however, more research is needed to confirm these findings.

Although there is evidence of a UL for vitamin E, it is unlikely that dietary intake would result in levels that may cause toxicity. With the highest range of intake being 25 to 31 mg/d, a UL of 1000 mg/d could only be reached by excessive consumption of supplements.

Vitamin B$_6$, commonly known as *pyridoxine*, is found in animal meats, cereals and grains, and other plant materials. At this time, although some populations of individuals may have inadequate intake, overall there does not seem to be a generalized problem with adequacy. In fact, greater concern surrounds individuals consuming too much of this vitamin. As a result, the UL is set at about 100 mg/d, roughly 100 times the requirement for adults under age 50. Historically, research reports of people consuming high levels of this vitamin demonstrated irreversible damage to their peripheral (limbs) nervous system.

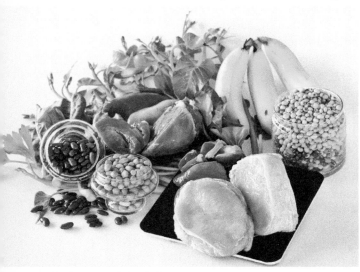
Food sources of vitamin B6

The coenzyme form of this vitamin, pyridoxal phosphate, has great significance in enhancing several different metabolic processes. Perhaps the most significant is the process of **transamination,** where unessential amino acids are formed from other amino acids. In addition, epinephrine, serotonin, and dopamine formation are dependent upon enzymes requiring pyridoxal phosphate. These neurotransmitters have been shown to have great significance upon neurological processes in the brain and are being evaluated for their impact upon peripheral processes as well. Although numerous other pathways may be dependent upon pyridoxal phosphate, the one most related to optimal health may be a pathway that leads to detoxification of homocysteine, resulting in a decreased risk for heart disease.

In addition to increased risk of heart disease as mentioned above, inadequate intake of vitamin B_6 can also lead to skin irritations, anemia, and neurological problems such as depression and confusion.

Transamination: A biochemical process whereby an amino group from a particular amino acid is transferred to a ketoacid, resulting in a new nonessential amino acid and a new ketoacid.

Minerals

Phosphorous is found in large quantities in the body, second only to calcium levels. Despite the large amount required for optimum bone and tooth formation, phosphorus deficiency is rarely seen. Most foods we eat have phosphorus in them in the form of phosphates, particularly foods high in protein. As a result we derive sufficient quantities from many common foods like meat, poultry, fish, and eggs. In addition to its important role in combining with calcium to form the matrix of bone and teeth, a small amount of total phosphorus is also used for functions outside of bone, including the structure of cell membranes and energy metabolism.

Due to the large amount of phosphorus in foods, finding individuals who are deficient in phosphorus is unusual. Occasionally, an individual may have insufficient body phosphorus due to taking high amounts of aluminum hydroxide antacids or due to alcoholism. The greater concern is that too much phosphorus may be consumed, particularly as phosphoric acid, an additive in soft drinks that could cause high losses of calcium from the body. Additionally, those with renal failure, who cannot dispose of phosphorus appropriately, may get toxicity resulting in low blood calcium, **tetany,** and excessive levels of calcium accumulating in the body's organs. These phenomena would only occur with levels beyond what we would normally consume, between 3000 and 4000 mg/d.

Zinc is a mineral that appears to be adequate in the U.S. diet, so we do not have a great concern regarding deficiency for the general population. Some evidence shows that this may not be true for select segments of the population, including pregnant women, young children, the elderly, and

Tetany: An uncontrollable twitching of a muscle, often due to mineral imbalance.

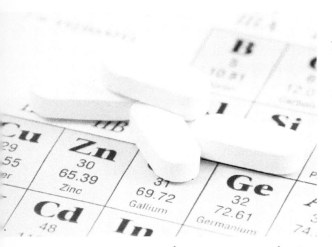

the poor. Zinc deficiency was, however, a major concern in places in the world where zinc was bound up by plant chemicals and made unavailable, particularly in many areas in the Middle East, where flatbreads are used. These breads are traditionally made in a way that does not use yeast. Yeast cells actually disable the plant materials that make zinc unavailable. The major plant chemical is called *phytic acid*, and although this problem has not occurred in the United States, we do need to be concerned that our plant sources of zinc are digestible. Zinc is present at the highest levels in protein foods, similar to phosphorus, but plant sources are also important for many to maintain dietary adequacy. In a subsequent chapter we discuss the pharmacological use of zinc, but our focus here is on its primary nutritional roles. From what is known at this time, zinc is important for growth and for maintaining the immune system. Evidence also supports the essentiality of zinc in taste perception, sperm production, and behavior and learning performance. When populations have been determined to be deficient, typically the deficiency signs are growth retardation in boys, an impaired immune response, and poor development or damage to the central nervous system.

Copper has not been seen to be deficient in either U.S. or global populations, as it is found in the diet in legumes, shellfish, nuts, and seeds. Many of us also receive a great deal of copper from our water supply as copper pipes provide this nutrient to our homes. Most of what we know about its role and deficiency is from experimental research and genetic disease. From the research literature, we have learned that copper is important to adequate functioning of our immune system and our antioxidant system. Copper also appears to be very significant in bone formation as well as the integrity of our cardiovascular system. In addition, it is a component of an enzyme called *ceruloplasmin*, which ensures that our bodies use iron appropriately. From studying the effects of Menkes syndrome, a rare childhood genetic disorder, it has been established that without copper being distributed to our tissues, we could not live. Specifically, the progressive cerebral degeneration in these children results in death by 2 years of age.

Although the UL for copper is set at 10 mg/d for adults, this is six times higher than the average intake by adult males. Although we do not anticipate seeing copper toxicity from the consumption of normal diets, toxicity could occur from overzealous consumption of supplements. Once again, we

Menkes Disease

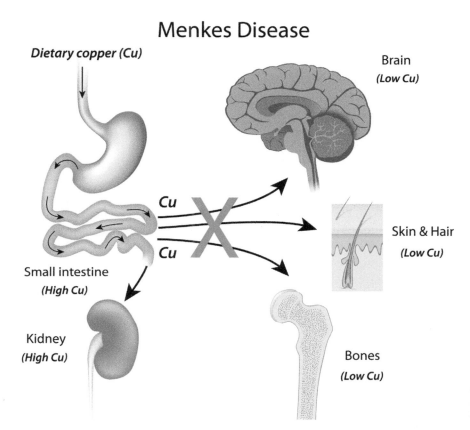

Dietary copper (Cu)

Brain
(Low Cu)

Cu

Cu

Skin & Hair
(Low Cu)

Small intestine
(High Cu)

Kidney
(High Cu)

Bones
(Low Cu)

Copper insufficiency due to Menke's Syndrome

have learned something about copper toxicity from a rare genetic disease. Wilson's disease can result in high levels of copper spreading throughout the body. It usually does not appear until the third decade of life and can be diagnosed by an unusual greenish color of the pupil of the eye. Wilson's disease can be treated with a drug that binds the copper and eliminates it from the body. No serious side effects appear to result from this condition.

Manganese is found in very small amounts in the human body, particularly in bones, joints, and metabolically active organs. Biochemically, it has been shown to be important for the activity of enzymes involved in the formation of connective tissue. Although the average intake (AI) for healthy people is between 2 and 3 mg we likely get sufficient amounts from our diets, particularly from grain products. There is an upper limit (UL) of 11 mg/d, but it is unlikely that an individual would consume such a high amount in their normal diets. Of course it is always possible to consume supplements at high levels to exceed the UL; however, the consequences have not been observed.

34 78.96
Se
Selenium

Selenium intake is generally adequate for most people living in the United States. There is some evidence of diseases that may occur in other countries where selenium intake may be inadequate. For a time, many professionals believed that higher levels of selenium would prevent cancer at various sites, but there is currently far less enthusiasm. Undoubtedly, selenium is important as part of our antioxidant system as part of the enzyme glutathione peroxidase. Selenium has been shown to be quite toxic, with symptoms such as brittle nails, nausea, and vomiting occurring with intake greater than 400 mg/d.

Trace elements such as molybdenum, nickel, silicon, vanadium, cobalt, and boron are suspected of having essentiality in humans, but it has not been conclusively demonstrated that they are required in our diets to maintain health. Most of the inferential evidence comes from animal studies and from isolated cells or tissues. Dietary deficiencies of these minerals are not known, and we are not yet sure of the level that would need to be consumed to result in toxicity. Perhaps the best evidence so far is for the essentiality of molybdenum, which does appear to be essential for the function of several enzymes. It is unlikely that deficiency would occur since it is found in many foods, including legumes, grain products, bread, leafy green vegetables, milk, and liver. As further research is accomplished, we will learn more about the other trace elements identified above.

Suggested Readings

Calvo MS, Uribarri J. Contributions to total phosphorus intake: All sources considered. *Semin Dial.* 2013; 26:54–61.

Gibson RS. A historical review of progress in the assessment of dietary zinc intake as an indicator of population zinc status. *Adv Nutr.* 2012; 3:772–82. doi: 10.2945/an.112.002287.

Simpson JL, Bailey LB, Pietrzik K, et al. Micronutrients and women of reproductive potential: Required dietary intake and consequences of dietary deficiency or excess. Part I—folate, vitamin B_{12}, vitamin B_6. *J Matern Fetal Neonatal Med.* 2010; 23:1323–43.

Ueland PM. Choline and betaine in health and disease. *J Inherit Metab Dis.* 2011; 34:3–15.

Vardi M, Levy NS, Levy AP. Vitamin E in the prevention of cardiovascular disease: The importance of proper patient selection. *J Lipid Res.* 2013; 54:2307–14.

HIGHLIGHT 6

Possible Functions of Phytochemicals Similar to Vitamin E and Implications for Dietary Supplementation

As discussed in this chapter, there are materials similar to vitamin E that differ only slightly from its structure. These phytochemicals include three other tocopherols and four tocotrienols. Some years ago, these similar compounds were evaluated for vitamin E activity and found to have much less activity than alpha-tocopherol. Recently, the Food and Nutrition Board determined that the term "vitamin E" would be limited only to the activity in food or supplements provided by alpha-tocopherol. Several recent reviews, however, have described the numerous studies demonstrating the anticarcinogenic properties of the other vitamin E–like phytochemicals upon breast, prostate, colorectal, and lung tumors in human populations, animal models, and cell culture.

The possible role of vitamin E in the form of alpha-tocopherol (AT) has been explored with respect to colon, rectal, and prostate tumor prevention with only moderately successful results. Numerous reviews, meta-analyses, and research papers have failed to provide evidence of a beneficial effect as a consequence of vitamin E (AT) treatment. Studies of human subjects as well as those using animal models have failed to show a reduction in tumors at all sites studied. In fact, these antioxidant nutrients are consumed at mega-doses, with probably more of a detrimental effect. Evidence suggests that pathways to anticarcinogenesis promoted by several of the vitamin E–like phytochemicals actually depend upon normal cellular oxidation processes and thus are hindered by excessive levels of cellular antioxidation, and that AT hinders the anticancer actions of gamma-tocopherol (GT) in an animal breast cancer model.

The effects of GT upon anticarcinogenesis has recently been a major focus because it is generally consumed in quantities higher than AT in the U.S. diet, and dietary consumption results in a reasonably high serum level of GT. While case-control and cohort studies strengthen the link between GT serum levels and a reduction in colorectal, lung, and prostate cancer, clinical intervention studies have not yet been accomplished for GT.

Studies of cultured tumor cells supplemented with various tocopherols have enabled researchers to evaluate possible mechanisms by which these phytochemicals exert their anticarcinogenic effects. These studies have resulted in some understanding of how GT and possibly other tocopherols may impact the growth of colon, breast, prostate, and lung cancer. The overall findings are that GT has been demonstrated to be an extremely potent inducer of apoptosis (cell death), as well as an inducer of cell cycle arrest in some cancer cells.

Dietary supplementation with either vitamin E (AT) or GT is not yet warranted for the general U.S. population. In the case of AT, overconsumption could lead to an increase in various cancers due to its interference upon GT's anticarcinogenic mechanisms. Although GT appears to be anticarcinogenic upon cultured tumor cells and in human case-control and cohort studies, the absence of clinical trials using GT supplements precludes a recommendation for dietary supplementation at this time.

Suggested Readings

This article is reprinted with the permission of the journal and was originally cited as:

Gerber, L.E. (2012) Physiobiochemical significance of vitamin E and other tocopherols in the U.S. diet: cancer promoters or preventers? J. Physiobiochem. Metab. 1,1-2.

Ju J, Picinich SC, Yang Z, Zhao Y, Suh N, et al. Cancer-preventive activities of tocopherols and tocotrienols. *Carcinogenesis.* 2010; 31:533–42.

Smolarek AK, Suh N. Chemopreventive activity of vitamin E in breast cancer: A focus on gamma- and delta-tocopherol. *Nutrients.* 2011; 3:962–86.

Wada S. Cancer preventive effects of vitamin E. *Curr Pharm Biotechnol.* 2010; 13:154–62.

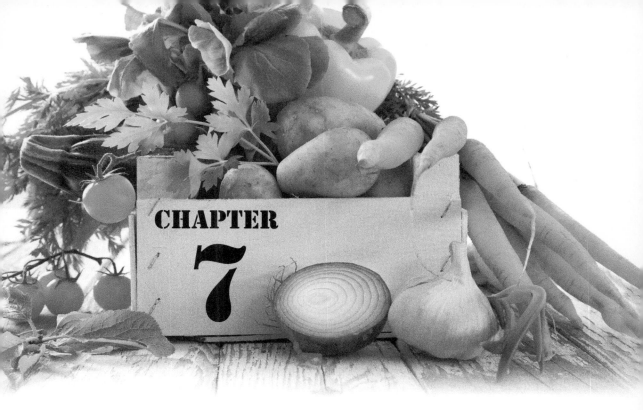

7

Concerns about Nutrients Often Consumed Excessively

Many of us, when left to consume as we please, coupled with the food industry's motivation to sell the consumer more of its product, often make food choices that can be dangerous for our health. I want to make one disclaimer at the beginning of this chapter: Some individuals may be more and some less genetically predisposed to have health issues when consuming excessive amounts of some of these nutrients. The Highlight that follows this chapter delves into some of these genetic issues that can affect the development of obesity and weight control.

Structures of various lipids

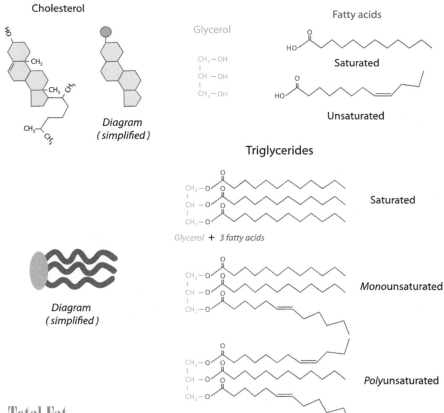

Cholesterol

Diagram
(simplified)

Glycerol

$CH_2 - OH$
$CH - OH$
$CH_2 - OH$

Fatty acids

Saturated

Unsaturated

Triglycerides

$CH_2 - O$
$CH - O$
$CH_2 - O$

Saturated

Glycerol + 3 fatty acids

Diagram
(simplified)

$CH_2 - O$
$CH - O$
$CH_2 - O$

Monounsaturated

$CH_2 - O$
$CH - O$
$CH_2 - O$

Polyunsaturated

Triglycerides: Common name for the chemical compound also known as a triacylglycerol. It is composed of a glycerol backbone, where each of the hydroxyl groups is esterified with a fatty acid.

Glycerol: The backbone of a triglyceride, composed of three carbons bonded together in a linear sequence, with each of the carbons having a hydroxyl group.

Monoglycerides: Common name for a monoacylglycerol, a lipid with only one fatty acid esterified to a glycerol backbone.

Total Fat

Total fat consumption, when excessive, can lead to excessive caloric intake. When we talk about fat calories, we are generally referring to the amount of triglycerides that are being consumed. Currently the USDA recommends a level of 20% to 35% of our dietary energy consumption coming from total fat. Later in this chapter we discuss specific types of triglycerides and their impact upon health. For the time, we only consider the total amount. In terms of kilocalories, triglycerides have been determined to provide 9 kilocalories per gram. This level is far greater than the kilocalories per gram for other energy-yielding macronutrients like protein, sugars, and starch, which provide about 4 kilocalories per gram. For brevity, we usually just use the common word "calories" rather than "kilocalories" to express the amount of energy provided by any of these nutrients.

    Triglycerides are absorbed from our diets through a rather complicated process, but basically they are broken down into their residual chemical components of **glycerol**, fatty acids, or **monoglycerides**, which re-form

Anatomy of a heart attack

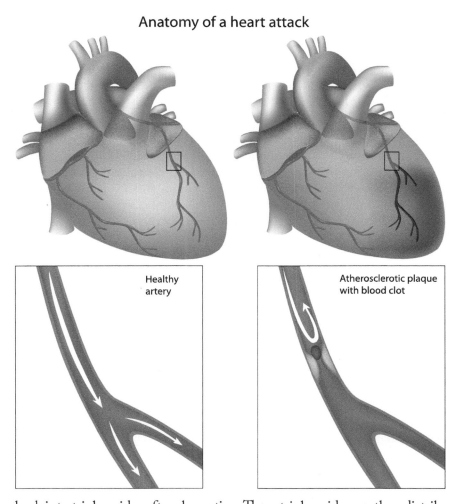

Healthy artery

Atherosclerotic plaque with blood clot

Formation of an atheroma and a resultant heart attack.

back into triglycerides after absorption. These triglycerides are then distributed for either energy or storage to the various organs of our body. Most of the storage occurs in cells called **adipocytes** located in our adipose tissue.

Wherever the fat is stored, it provides, in theory, reserves of energy for times when inadequate energy is being consumed.

For many years, it was believed that the total amount of fat in the diet was responsible for the formation of **atheromas** and therefore responsible for greater levels of cardiovascular disease in those who consumed large amounts of fat. It was also believed that greater fat intake was responsible for greater cancer incidence at many sites in the body. Although advances in scientific research have shown that the specific types of fat consumed have a greater impact upon the development of cardiovascular disease,

Adipocytes: The technical name for fat cells, those cells that are biologically active in our adipose tissue that either store or release fat.

Atheromas: A mass of plaque consisting of various lipids and other cellular debris that generally obstructs blood flow in our arteries. Typically the cause of atherosclerosis.

when a person eats an inordinate amount of fat, usually the fats that cause the most problems are consumed in high amounts as well.

Contemporary research has also demonstrated that total fat intake probably does not directly contribute to most incidence of cancer, except for colon cancer. When fat is consumed, a greater amount of bile acids are secreted, which can induce the colon to develop cancerous cells. At this time there is no scientific evidence to demonstrate that fat intake results in cancers at other sites, although researchers continue to investigate whether there is also a link to breast and prostate cancer.

Also, there is an indirect link between high consumption of fat, which usually results in higher consumption of calories and results in deposits in the adipocytes, and disease. Recent studies suggest that accumulation of high amounts of fat in the abdominal area may result in greater potential for the development of diabetes, hypertension, cardiovascular disease, and possibly some types of cancer. Further work is needed before recommendations can be made. It should also be pointed out that abdominal adipose can come from excess intake of protein and carbohydrates.

Double bonds: The connection between some elements that are part of a molecule, which consists of two bonds between the elements, as compared to a single bond, which has only one connection. Double bonds are generally less stable to oxidation than single bonds.

Saturated fats are those that do not have any **double bonds** between their carbons and are fully "saturated" with hydrogen atoms. Saturated fats are typically solids at room temperature and make up the composition of butter and most traditional shortenings like beef tallow and lard. Although suspected for some time, scientists eventually determined that the high amounts of saturated fat in high-fat diets were the predominant factor in encouraging cardiovascular disease, since the presence of saturated fat in arteries makes them less capable of movement when they are needed for proper blood flow.

There are material advantages to saturated fats for both the industry and the consumer. Because of their lack of double bonds, they are more resistant to oxidative damage, which enables the manufacturer to have a product with increased shelf life. This can be passed on to the consumer at a reduced price due to the diminished cost of stocking the grocery store with the product. In our homes, these products also can be stored longer without spoilage and do not generally need to be refrigerated.

Trans-monounsaturated fat: A type of fatty acid, sometimes found in nature, but occurring in high amounts after polyunsaturated oils have been treated chemically to result in monounsaturated fat. The fatty acids have a trans configuration around the remaining double bond, meaning that the hydrogen atoms of the two adjacent carbon structures are on the opposite sides.

"Trans" monounsaturated fat is a specific type of fat that rarely originates naturally in the food that we consume, but instead is a product of food processing. This type of fat differs from the naturally occurring "cis"-monounsaturated fat that is common in many foods.

Until the 1940s, trans monounsaturated fat was not a significant component of our diets, but as butter and other shortenings became in short supply due to the deprivations of World War II, it became necessary to produce substitutes. Food chemists turned to a known reaction that

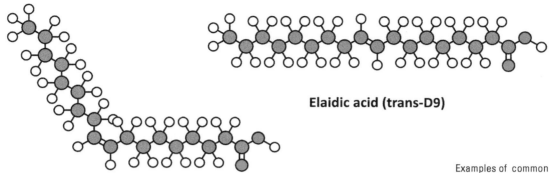

Elaidic acid (trans-D9)

Oleic acid (cis-D9)

Examples of common "cis" and "trans" fatty acids

could alter **polyunsaturated fats** to monounsaturated fats. Unfortunately, the reaction cannot be controlled adequately to produce only cis-monounsaturated fats but instead produces an approximately equal amount of trans monounsaturated fats. At the time this process was begun, it was not known that the trans fats would have harmful effects upon the human body, and manufacturers were delighted—as were consumers—as they now could produces substitutes for butter and shortenings such as lard or beef tallow. Not for many decades did researchers begin to determine that these trans fats were so structurally similar to saturated fats that they resulted in increased risk for cardiovascular disease.

Because of the enormity of evidence linking trans saturated fats to cardiovascular disease, the FDA has recently required all food companies to label their products with the amount of trans fat in a serving of food. This requirement has resulted in the voluntary removal of much of the trans fat that was previously being used in many foods. These types of fats have been traditionally used in snack foods and fast foods. In the latter case, it has been due indirectly to the deep frying used for French fries and other foods that are fried in highly trans monounsaturated fats. Many municipalities have actually begun to place bans on the use of these fats in restaurants. Not surprisingly, this will likely result in higher prices to consumers, since this change will result in greater cost to restaurants due to the shorter amount of time these substitutes can be used. Additionally, the polyunsaturated fat substitutes have a greater tendency to form carcinogenic materials when heated. The answer to this conundrum is beyond the scope of this text, but future research will enable us to make appropriate decisions.

Cholesterol, although an essential component of cellular membranes and critical for the synthesis of numerous bioactive molecules, is not an essential nutrient. Although cholesterol is a very large molecule, most cells are able to manufacture it from smaller molecules. Initially, research

Polyunsaturated fats: Fats generally found as liquids at room temperature and characterized by having fatty acids with two or more double bonds.

Structure of LDL and HDL lipoproteins.

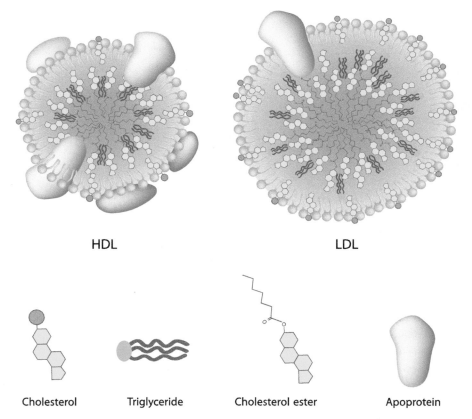

HDL   LDL

Cholesterol   Triglyceride   Cholesterol ester   Apoprotein

Plaque: Often used similarly to the term atheroma, as they are collections of various lipids and cellular debris that accumulate on the intima of arteries.

Low-density lipoprotein (LDL): A lipoprotein particle produced in the blood that is high in cholesterol and deposited in various organs as well as arteries.

High-density lipoprotein (HDL): A lipoprotein particle produced in the liver that is low in cholesterol and high in specific proteins, capable of removing cholesterol from the body for disposal.

scientists suspected that cholesterol intake was the significant factor in the development of cardiovascular disease. The research was based upon the evaluation of individuals who had heart attacks early in life. As a result, it was erroneously concluded that the excess intake of cholesterol resulted in cardiovascular events. It was later determined that these individuals suffered from a genetic disease that prevented them from disposing of excess cholesterol. The excess intake resulted in the cholesterol depositing in **plaque** in their arteries, which resulted in blockage of blood flow. Healthy individuals are normally able to dispose of reasonable amounts of excessive cholesterol and also decrease the amount of cholesterol typically produced by the cells of the liver. Current research has led us to understand how cholesterol is distributed to cells and organs through a lipoprotein called **low-density lipoprotein (LDL)** and can be removed for disposal by **high-density lipoprotein (HDL)**. We now understand that some people cannot adjust to high levels of cholesterol in their diet due to genetic reasons, but most people are unaware of their genetic predispositions. Although looking at one's relatives may give a hint as to genetic predispositions, there is no substitute for genetic testing to be certain. As a result of most people not knowing their genetic status, intake of not more than 300 mg/d is recommended to prevent cardiovascular disease in susceptible individuals.

Sugars and Starches

Sugars and starches are likely overconsumed, as opposed to the carbohydrate family of fiber that we underconsume. In particular, the major health concern is the amount of added sugars we consume on average per day, which is about 120 grams. The sugars found naturally in foods are not included in this total, as the natural sugar **fructose** is primarily found in fruits. We look at the bigger picture here and understand that fruits are a superb source of fiber and many micronutrients.

Fructose and other sugars provide the necessary energy to cells after they are transformed to glucose in the liver. The other sugars found naturally in our diet include lactose in milk and maltose in sprouting grains, but the amounts are low and do not contribute substantially to our overall intake. **Starches** are also a large component of grains, fruits, and vegetables, all of which we need in abundance. Here, too, the natural starch is easily broken down in the digestive tract to its residual glucose units. **Glucose** can also be stored in the liver as the complex carbohydrate **glycogen,** which can be used when blood sugar is not adequate. So, in brief, we get more than enough sugar for energy use and storage from the foods we should be eating, from the fructose as well as the starches found naturally in these foods.

Fructose: A simple monosaccharide sugar, commonly found in fruits or as part of the table sugar (sucrose) molecule, sweeter than most other sugars.

Starches: Various collections of glucose molecules in large chains; some may be linear where others may be branched. Generally each plant food has its own particular starch.

Glucose: A simple monosaccharide sugar, not usually found by itself, but part of all of the common disaccharides—including sucrose, mannose, and lactose—as well as the sugar that makes up starch chains.

Glycogen: A storage form of glucose chains in the human and animal body, found as a branched-chain collection. Typically accumulates in muscles and liver.

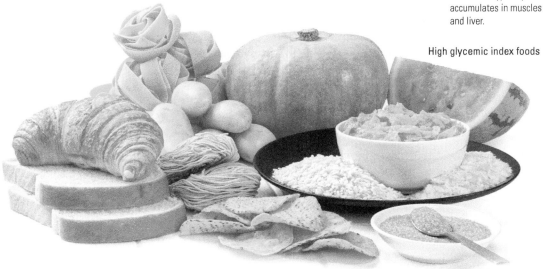

High glycemic index foods

Low glycemic index foods.

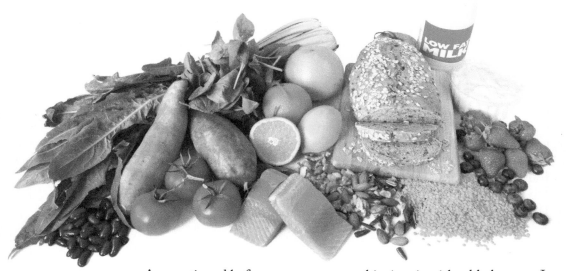

As mentioned before, our concern at this time is with added sugars. In fact, recommendations have suggested that not more than 10% to 25% of our total energy consumed in a day should come from added sugars. In the future, the issue of added starches may need to be addressed, but it has not been determined if these are detrimental to our overall health. Numerous studies have shown that excessive consumption of added sugars do have a detrimental effect upon our health in several ways. These include the development of diabetes and coronary heart disease, as well as obesity. We explore the factors underlying obesity and weight control in the Highlight that follows this chapter.

In order to understand the relationship of excess sugar or starch consumption to health, we have to understand the concepts of glycemic index and glycemic load. The glycemic index of a food is generally proportional to the food's capacity to increase the levels of the blood sugar glucose and the hormone insulin. These values are compared to a standard, which can either be glucose or white bread. Whichever standard is used is assigned a value of 100%. The test food will be given a value compared to the standard, based upon its ability to raise blood glucose and insulin.

Glycemic load is determined by multiplying the glycemic index of a food by the grams of carbohydrate in a typical serving of that particular food. Research from several laboratories has confirmed that foods with high levels of added sugar and carbohydrates result in high glycemic indices and high glycemic loads. Other factors may also influence these values for a given food, including the amount of fiber present as well as protein and fat. Some of the foods with a high glycemic index include white bread, potatoes, bagels, Cheerios, corn flakes, and Coca-Cola. Those demonstrated to have a low glycemic index include beans, raw apples, tomato juice, lentils, and All-Bran cereal. Other foods tested have values between the lowest and the highest glycemic index foods.

Various agencies have determined the appropriate ranges of intake for carbohydrates (including sugar and starch). The USDA has determined the DRI to be 45% to 65% of the energy requirement, with a RDA of 130 g/d. The FDA has determined the daily value (DV) for carbohydrates to be 60% of energy intake, with a recommended intake of 300 g/d.

Energy-Yielding Nutrients

Energy-yielding nutrient recommendations have been debated extensively. We have already seen much progress for recommended fat and carbohydrate intake. Protein intake is often excessive but for some may be inadequate, as discussed in chapter 4. Prevention of obesity and appropriate energy control is extremely important and are discussed in the Highlight that follows this chapter. Although there are DRI ranges for energy-yielding macronutrients set by the USDA, it is easy to surpass one's caloric needs by eating at the higher percentages of these ranges. Even if consumption is moderate, inadequate activity can result in an imbalance of excessive calories, resulting in weight gain.

Sodium Chloride (Salt)

Sodium chloride (salt) intake has been excessive in the typical U.S. diet for some time. Ironically, a historical value has been placed on salt due to its global absence. Recent archaeological findings suggest that salt may have been one of the most valued commodities in various regions of the world due to its limited presence. In fact, many of the great sea voyages centuries ago had as their goal to find sources of salt. Even in today's world, we find animals living in the wild that are unable to get enough salt to function properly, and we provide salt licks in the forest for them.

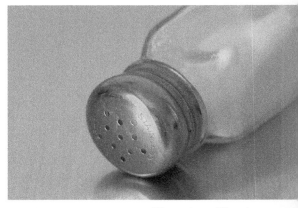

We may have different ways of consuming salt today, but our desire to consume it is still the same

How did we get to our current situation of salt overconsumption, and just how bad is it? Part of the reason for overconsumption is that salt is currently inexpensive and greatly available in our country, and we have acquired a taste for it. Part of our abundant use is due to the tradition of sprinkling salt on our foods or incorporating it into the foods we eat. Another factor has been commercial food companies' use of salt to either mask the taste of foods that are not palatable due to food processing or to enhance the taste of a food. Currently, we are more consumed with sodium intake, although the chloride component of the molecule is being explored as to its effects. In the recent results of the NHANES III study, adult men were found to consume about 4 g/d of sodium, while adult women consume about 3 g/d of sodium. Although there is no established RDA for sodium, there is an established AI. It varies with age, declining from 1.5 to 1.2 g/d as a person matures from young adulthood to older age. In fact, the Food and Nutrition Board has set a UL of 2.3 g/d. Clearly many of us are consuming more than is recommended, and a significant number are consuming toxic levels.

High blood pressure (hypertension): A condition typified by having higher than normal blood pressure both when the heart is contracting to pump blood and also during the interval between the heart's contraction to pump the blood.

The main reason we are concerned about excessive salt intake is that sodium encourages higher amounts of fluid to flow into the cardiovascular system. These higher levels result in a need for the heart to beat harder to push this increased amount of fluid through the system and ultimately results in higher blood pressure. Another cause of **high blood pressure** due to excessive salt intake may be the elevation of angiotensin in the blood, which elevates blood pressure. In most people this is a transient phenomena that occurs primarily if blood pressure becomes somewhat low; however, in others the phenomena becomes persistent and results in continuous elevation of blood pressure. Research studies have shown a genetic and age-related component to the predisposition of high blood pressure. For instance, African Americans have a high prevalence, as do older Americans. In addition to its known association with high blood pressure

Although salt is not solely to blame, it is a factor in our nation's overall hypertensive crisis.

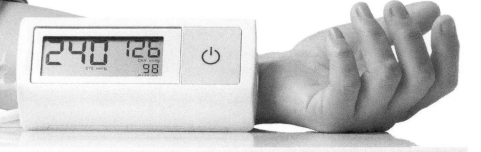

(hypertension), salt also is a deterrent to maintenance of bone calcium. High salt intake encourages urinary losses of calcium, one of the potential factors in preventing optimum bone maintenance. In addition, high salt intake has been associated with mucosal damage and gastric cancer.

Perhaps the most compelling evidence associating salt intake with hypertension is the thirty-two-country Intersalt Cooperative Research Group Study of more than 10,000 men and women. Despite only a weak finding for the relationship of hypertension to higher excretion of salt, the study did show that salt restriction resulted in lower amounts of hypertension in general, but more specifically was a factor for older individuals.

Suggested Readings

Aller EE, Abete I, Astrup A et al. Starches, sugars and obesity. *Nutrients.* 2011; 3:341–69.

Ganguly R, Pierce GN. Trans fat involvement in cardiovascular disease. *Mol Nutr Food Res.* 2012; 56:1090–6.

Ha SK. Dietary salt intake and hypertension. *Electrolyte Blood Press.* 2014; 12:7–18.

Schwab U, Lauritzen L, Tholstrup T, et al. Effect of the amount and type of dietary fat on cardiovascular risk factors and risk of developing type 2 diabetes, cardiovascular disease, and cancer: a systematic review. *Food Nutr Res.* 2014; 58. doi: 10.342/fnr.v58.25145.

HIGHLIGHT 7

Obesity and Weight Control

The major purposes of this highlight are to explain how obesity arises and how we define it, to focus on the problems it causes, and to discuss some possible solutions. This highlight is not meant to be a comprehensive review of all the literature in the field, but rather an applied approach toward handling a serious and increasingly common problem. Overweight and obesity have been growing at an alarming rate since the 1990s. Around that time, most states in the United States had an obesity rate of less than 15% of their population. The current U.S. obesity rate is 27.7%, according to survey results released in 2014. This rate is higher than the rate for the previous year, which shows an alarming trend. Similarly, the same survey indicated that only 35% of those living in the United States were of normal weight. Unfortunately, obesity appears to be highest for some of our most vulnerable groups, including African Americans, Latinos, and those living on low incomes. Other groups appear to be women and those living in the southern and midwestern sections of the country.

How Does Obesity Arise?

The easy answer is that body fat begins to accrue to levels higher than appropriate when our energy consumption becomes greater than our energy use. Although some of us "live to eat," in reality we all must "eat to live." When we consume as many calories as we are using to live, then we will not increase our adipose stores. We need energy for three purposes: (1) required internal bodily activity such as maintaining our body temperature, the beating of our heart, and general metabolic activity; (2) most obviously, the physical activities that are part of our daily routine, whether it is the minimum required to function or a much higher level due to voluntary exercise; and (3) energy used to digest the foods we consume and absorb the resulting nutrients. Under normal circumstances we all get hungry and desire to eat. Those of us who are attuned to our body's responses feel satiation as a result of consuming enough food and refrain from eating more. Also, most people experience satiety after a meal and delay their eating of another meal. These responses are not learned but are innately part of our biological responses.

Unfortunately, because we can override our biological responses, we often eat more during a meal and eat more frequently than is needed. It is very easy to finish a meal and leave room for dessert. Likewise, snacking behavior is extremely common—perhaps due to boredom or just the availability of tasty foods.

Genetics likely plays a significant part in whether individuals have a predisposition toward overweight and obesity. There are approximately 100 genes that are being considered for influencing weight. Some of those genes appear to influence appetite, while others influence the way energy is used in the body. Proteins like ghrelin and leptin have been explored but do not seem to individually be the silver bullet. Perhaps more research will enable us to determine those genes that influence our propensity for obesity. Some of the best research in this field emanates from studies of populations that originated together but currently are separate—one with high rates of obesity, the other without. The Pima Native American Studies are among some of the best.

How Do We Define Overweight and Obesity?

Two important concepts need to be addressed here. First, several different metrics can be used to define overweight and obesity. Second, the difference between being overweight and obese is more than semantic. In terms of metrics, we have three different measurements: body mass index (BMI), percentage body fat, and waist circumference. BMI is commonly used for surveys of large groups of individuals or for single individuals when it is too tedious to do a more rigorous procedure. BMI is equal to a person's weight/mass in kilograms, divided by their height in meters squared. For instance if a woman weighs 50 kilograms (about 110 pounds) and is 1.5 meters (about 5 feet) tall, her BMI would be $50 / (1.5)^2$, which would be about 22. Based upon numerous individuals, we assign normalcy to those between 18.5 and 24.9. Individuals with a BMI between 25 and 29.9 are considered overweight. Those over 30 are considered obese. We differentiate between overweight and obesity even in this simple calculation.

Far more complicated are the techniques for determining percentage body fat. Several strategies are used in practice and research. The most common and probably the one in use the longest is the fat-fold measurement.

For this strategy, a skilled observer measures the fat-fold thicknesses of various parts of the subject. These have been verified to correlate with percentage body composition after transformation using various equations. Other more recent techniques include measuring the relationship between weight of a subject under water and in air, the resistance of a low electrical current through a subject's body, placing the subject in a sealed chamber and measuring their displacement of air, and finally the DEXA (Dual Energy X-ray Absorptiometry), which actually is accomplished by applying two different low-dose X-rays across key parts of a subject's body. All of these, through a variety of scientifically based equations, will approximate the percentage fat of an individual. Our criteria for overfatness for young men is not more than 22% fat, while for young women our criteria is not more than 32% body fat. For those at least 40 years old, we use 25% and 35%, respectively, for men and women.

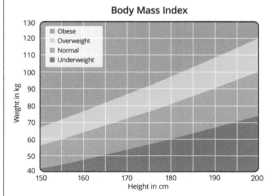

Body Mass Index

The most recent evaluations are based upon measuring waist circumference. It is currently believed that the most injurious adipose stores are those in the abdominal area, so we consider overfat as a waist circumference of 35 inches or more for adult women and 40 inches or more for adult men.

What problems do overweight and obesity cause? Some of the problems that may be associated with overweight and obesity are disease-related. For instance, cardiovascular disease may be brought about by the high blood cholesterol and hypertension that ensues with an abundance of body fat. In addition, diabetes mellitus type 2 may be brought on by the insulin resistance accompanying too much body fat. Even various types of cancer, particularly those resulting from an abundance of estrogen like breast and ovarian cancer, may be due to too much body fat. Some of these disorders as well as others may be linked to the discovery that too much body fat results in inflammation. It should also be noted that the initial research in this area seems to suggest a strong correlation with abdominal obesity.

Other problems emanating from overweight and obesity are more of a psychological and social nature. No doubt an elevation in body fat often leads to low self-esteem. In addition, although it is not condonable, discrimination for employment and other purposes is a problem that overweight and obese people may face.

What Possible Solutions Are There for the Person Who Needs to Lose Body Fat?

Of course, modern medicine has developed surgical procedures and medicines to enable some individuals to reduce their body fat. Since the American Medical Association has recognized obesity as a disease, physicians may either perform procedures or prescribe medicines for those who are obese. Remember, obesity is generally defined as a BMI of 30 or over. So far, surgical procedures have either involved removal of fat cells or reducing the size of the stomach (bariatric surgery). Liposuction is a surgical procedure

Adjustable Gastric Band (Lap Band)

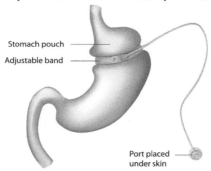

Stomach pouch

Adjustable band

Port placed
under skin

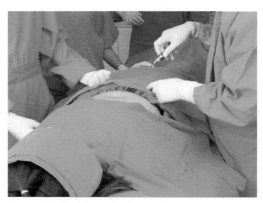

An actual liposuction procedure.

that can be used to selectively remove fat cells in a stepwise process to bring the person's weight to normalcy. Over the last several decades, surgeons have been trying to reduce food intake by procedures related to the gastrointestinal tract, with the gastric bypass and gastric banding procedures currently being used. Both procedures reduce the size of the stomach. None of these procedures can guarantee that obesity will not recur, as individuals can still find ways to overeat and regain their adipose stores.

The most current pharmacologic treatments include two different strategies. The drug orlistat reduces the amount of fat that the small intestine can absorb. The drugs phentermine and diethylpropion reduce food intake by altering neurotransmitter levels in the brain to mimic a feeling of fullness. Both of these drugs, as most do, have side effects. In the case of orlistat, the unabsorbed fat can result in gas and frequent bowel movements. In the case of drugs that influence neurotransmitters, they often result in high blood pressure and insomnia.

Those who practice nutrition and dietetics still believe that weight reduction can be accomplished more gradually through eating smaller portions of food at meals, increasing exercise, and practicing behaviors that encourage a feeling of higher self-esteem when weight is lost.

Suggested Readings

Kelley GA, Kelley KS. Effects of exercise in the treatment of overweight and obese children and adolescents: A systematic review of meta-analyses. *J Obes.* 2013; 2013:783103.

Leidy HJ. Increased dietary protein as a dietary strategy to prevent and/or treat obesity. *Mo Med.* 2014; 111:54–8.

Meany G, Conceicao E, Mitchell JE. Binge eating, binge eating disorder, and loss of control eating: Effects on weight outcomes after bariatric surgery. *Eur Eat Disord Rev.* 2014; 22:87–91.

Munsters MJ, Saris WH. Body weight regulation and obesity: Dietary strategies to improve the metabolic profile. *Annu Rev Food Sci Technol.* 2014; 5:39–51.

Vetter ML, Amaro A, Volger S. Nutritional management of type 2 diabetes mellitus and obesity and pharmacologic therapies to facilitate weight loss. *Postgrad Med.* 2014; 126:139–52.

Pharmacological Value of Common Nutrients, Herbals, and Phytochemicals

Until this chapter we have been presenting the value of nutrients as they are found naturally in the foods we eat or from small supplements that intend to substitute for our inability to obtain some of these nutrients from our normal diet. In this chapter we discuss the impact that some nutrients, herbals and phytochemicals may have when they are consumed at levels far beyond what we would normally find in our diets. These nutrients, herbals and phytochemicals are commonly provided like other medicinal materials—in pill or capsule form—and in the cases identified seem to provide benefits different from those obtained when these same substances are consumed at dietary levels.

Nutrients

Ascorbic acid has probably been the most discussed and the most consumed pharmacological dietary supplement. Initially it was believed that ascorbic acid could prevent colds and also cure numerous types of cancers. The data obtained, unfortunately, suffered from several serious methodological errors. In the case of cold prevention, the early studies did not use a **double-blind** or placebo experimental model. In other words, the subjects, the investigators, or both knew that the subjects were receiving ascorbic acid, and no placebo controls—individuals receiving pills or capsules devoid of ascorbic acid—were used. The problem with these results is that the subjects and investigators knew that ascorbic acid was being provided and the results were prejudiced by that knowledge. We know that the power of suggestion encourages people to self-report positively, and we also know that investigators are more inclined to report positive results when they are aware of a treatment being used on subjects. When these same experiments were repeated with the double-blind and placebo design, the results were not duplicated; ascorbic acid did not prevent colds. It was, however, concluded that at pharmacological levels, ascorbic acid taken at the beginning of and throughout a cold diminished the number of days that the

Double-blind:
An experimental design where neither the experimental nor control groups are aware of whether they are receiving a treatment and the investigators are also unaware of which subjects are in a treatment or control group.

Vitamin C supplements are consumed by many people.

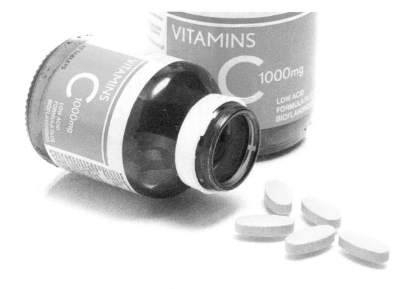

subjects felt uncomfortable. The current belief is that vitamin C functions as an antihistamine, similar to other antihistamines that are available by prescription or over the counter.

As for the possible impact of consuming high levels of ascorbic acid on the cure for various cancers, the original research was primarily clinical and anecdotal, as the subjects were patients with various types of cancer who had already had chemotherapy, radiation therapy, or surgery and were hoping that they might find a cure after being unsuccessful trying these other strategies. The results suggested that some patients were "cured" of their cancers, but again there were no double-blind or placebo designs, so the results are not meaningful. When vitamin C was used in clinical trials as a possible cure for various cancers, no such effect was seen. Currently, the only possible interaction with cancer for high levels of vitamin C may be to prevent gastrointestinal cancer.

At this point, research demonstrates that, for most people, the consumption of 500 mg/d of vitamin C will not be harmful, although there are no clear benefits. Unfortunately, those consuming 2000 mg/d or more may experience toxicity, including diarrhea, nausea, and heartburn.

Niacin has been used pharmacologically for several purposes. At levels of up to 6 g/d, nicotinic acid seemed to reduce high blood cholesterol by decreasing levels of LDL and increasing levels of HDL. It was hypothesized that niacin reduces fat breakdown and causes a decrease in liver synthesis and secretion of very-low-density lipoprotein (VLDL). Recent clinical trials do not support this claim.

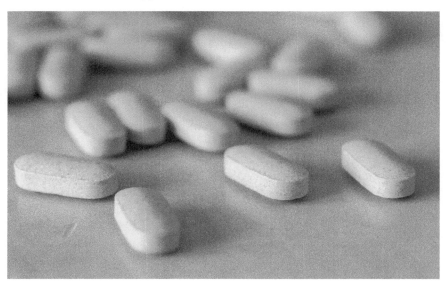

Niacin is one of the many B vitamin supplements consumed at high levels believed to improve health.

Another use of nicotinic acid has been to exaggerate the lines of the arterio-venous system as it appears on the skin and also to produce a niacin "flush." Some bodybuilders use this practice, particularly when they are competing or having a photo session. Although this is really a toxic effect of nicotinic acid, the effects are short-lived and do not cause permanent damage. In fact, those taking nicotinic acid for LDL cholesterol reduction also experience the niacin flush. Nicotinic acid causes a vasodilation response, which is why people experience swelling of the arteries and veins as well as a flushing of the skin.

Omega-3 fatty acids were discussed in Chapter 3. Recent evidence suggests that not only do we need these fatty acids to maintain normal health but they can also be used pharmacologically with benefits. In particular, physicians can now prescribe a purified omega-3 fatty acid capsule for reducing high blood triglycerides. High amounts can also be purchased over the counter, but the purity has come into question. High consumption of omega-3 fatty acids can also reduce blood clotting. This discovery was originally made among the Greenland Eskimos, who had a very low rate of heart attack, but numerous issues with hemorrhaging. This supplement can be very helpful for those who are at risk for blood clotting, which can lead to heart attack, stroke, or peripheral arterial clotting. Although it is not available by prescription for this purpose, many people buy supplements and use these rather than other anticlotting drugs, such as Coumadin.

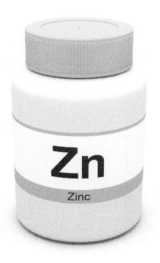

Zinc was discussed in chapter 6 as one of the nutrients that is typically consumed at about adequate levels in most diets, but generally not at excessive levels. Recently, consumers began to purchase zinc lozenges, sprays, and tablets because of some evidence that zinc has an impact on the survival and proliferation of viruses, like the rhinovirus, responsible for the common cold. Although the results are far from clear, zinc appears to have some impact in preventing colds when the person is first exposed to the virus. Some people believe that those who respond favorably may have been zinc inadequate before they took the supplements. In any event, the most recent studies suggest that the amount of zinc provided by lozenges does not appear to be adequate to make an impact on the susceptibility or effects of colds. Taking tablets appears to provide adequate amounts of zinc, but people taking zinc in this way should be careful about toxicity as the adult UL for zinc is 40 mg/d, and many supplements are provided in 50 mg tablets. Daily intake of

Currently, it is believed that zinc supplements may reduce cold susceptibility for some.

these levels over time can result in a copper deficiency as well as numbness and weakness. Some companies have introduced intranasal sprays and gels, which often result in a permanent loss of smell in some individuals.

Calcium was discussed in chapter 3 because it is commonly found in inadequate levels in many diets and is important in bone formation. Recent studies using pharmacological levels of calcium have demonstrated that there are fewer colorectal adenomas (cancer sites) in individuals consuming higher levels of calcium. One study did demonstrate a greater risk of prostate cancer for those men consuming the higher levels of calcium.

Herbals

Herbal materials have been used for medicinal purposes for millennia. Quite a few are currently popular for their possible curative and preventative properties. Most herbals are found in plants that are not generally consumed for their nutrient content. Herbal materials are regulated by the Food and Drug Administration but are not allowed to have health claims on the labels. One of the most serious concerns is the purity of the herbal materials sold, as no regulatory agency oversees their quality. This section of the chapter discusses commonly available herbal materials as well as one plant.

Numerous herbal supplements in capsule form are now available.

Echinacea has been suggested to be a deterrent to colds, upper respiratory infections, and flulike symptoms. The biological basis for these effects is reported to be a boosting of the immune system by one or more active agents in the plant. The capsules that are sold are composed of the roots, flowers, and leaves from the echinacea plant, which resembles the common daisy. The purveyors of the product recommend consuming between 500 and 1000 mg/d for optimal effect.

Numerous effects have been reported with the consumption of *garlic*. These include a reduction of blood pressure, blood lipids, blood glucose, and blood clotting, which should be helpful in many disease states if true. In addition, garlic has also been suggested to be an antioxidant, an anticarcinogen, and an immune system–enhancing agent. Recommended intakes by the manufacturers range from 600 to 900 mg/d of powdered garlic, generally in capsule form.

Gingko biloba also has many purported attractive attributes, including improved blood flow, particularly in the brain. It comes from the leaves of a tall tree with gray-colored bark, originally indigenous to China. Numerous active ingredients found in this plant may have a role

Vasodilation: Expansion of the vessels of the circulatory system to allow for greater volumes of blood passage through them.

in inducing peripheral **vasodilation**, reducing blood clotting, and antioxidation, and clinically significant effects have been seen with dose levels of 120 mg/d, generally as extracts in capsule form.

True *ginseng* is derived from the root of shade plants native to Korea and China, but there are also some species in the United States and other places (typically without the same bioactivity). Ginseng is purported to reduce fatigue and improve stamina, and may also be an anticarcinogen and an antioxidant. Recommended intakes range from 100 to 300 mg/d of the extract.

St. John's Wort has been suggested to inhibit neurotransmitter metabolism, resulting in an improvement in depression and anxiety. It is a perennial herb that produces golden yellow flowers. The flowers are dried and extracted for bioactive materials. Proponents of St. John's Wort have suggested a recommended dose of about 1000 mg/d.

Phenolic: A chemical structure derived from phenol, an aromatic crystalline compound, often with biological activity.

Phytochemicals

Phytochemicals in foods were discussed to some extent in Highlight 5, particularly some of the **phenolic** materials and carotenoids found in foods. In this chapter, I focus on some specific phytochemicals found in plants that are often sold as supplements, including curcumin, quercetin, and resveratrol.

Curcumin, extracted from the common spice turmeric and used in curry powder, has been suggested to have tremendous health benefits when consumed as an extract in capsules. The extract is typically taken from the root of the turmeric plant. Curcumin is a polyphenol that has been shown to have antioxidant and anti-inflammatory properties. In addition, some have shown that it may also reduce blood clot formation. Suggested doses range from 1000 to 1500 mg/d. These levels would not be possible to consume as part of a normal dietary intake.

Curcumin is extracted from curry powder and believed to have antioxidant and anti-inflammatory properties.

Quercetin can be extracted from a wide variety of plants, none of which are part of our habitual diet. Structurally, it is a **flavonoid**, and a variety of evidence from animal models and cell studies shows its health value. Suggested uses are as a substitute for other drugs used for the prevention of cardiovascular disease and also as an antihypertensive agent. More recently, an animal model was used to demonstrate its value in the treatment of obesity, and studies have also recently demonstrated its anticarcinogenic

Flavonoid: A chemical structure of numerous plant materials with a flavone component, many of which have biological activity.

properties. Although the reports are somewhat anecdotal, quercetin has been suggested for chronic prostate inflammation. Although most supplements are supplied in 250 mg capsules, suggested consumption levels are about 1000 mg/d.

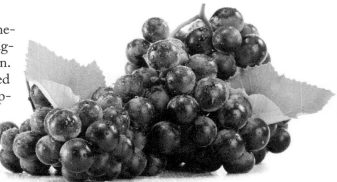

Resveratrol can be found in either grapes or grape juice.

Resveratrol is probably the most controversial of the phytochemicals suggested to have health effects due to its origin in red wine and grape juice. The controversy began due to the finding that consumption of red wine had a cardiovascular protective effect. Subsequent research did not confirm that red wine was the only alcoholic beverage with this effect, but rather all alcoholic beverages were demonstrated to have similar effects. It is now believed that ethanol (alcohol) has its own effect upon individuals generally above age 50 that results in a reduction of cardiovascular risk. Although resveratrol is found in red wine, it is also found in red grape juice as well as the skin of red grapes and raspberries. Most people will not likely consume enough resveratrol to obtain its benefits on a normal diet. Resveratrol is also a flavonoid and is suggested to have benefits in inhibiting cancer growth and reducing inflammation, as seen in animal studies. Most supplements usually have no more than 500 mg per capsule; however, to mimic the effects on cancer and inflammation seen in these studies, people would need to take 2000 mg/d of resveratrol.

Suggested Readings

Owens C, Baergen R, Puckett D. Online sources of herbal product information. *Am J Med.* 2014; 127:109–15.

Prasad AS. Zinc: Role in immunity, oxidative stress and chronic inflammation. *Curr Opin Clin Nutr Metab Care.* 2009; 12:646–52.

Salvamani S, Gunasekaran B, Shaharuddin NA, et al. Antiartherosclerotic effects of plant flavonoids. *Biomed Res Intl.* 2014; Article ID 480258.

Swanson D, Block R, Mousa SA. Omega-3 fatty acids EPA and DHA: Health benefits throughout life. *Adv Nutr.* 2012; 3:1–7.

Tiwari V, Khokar M. Mechanism of action of anti-hypercholesterolemia drugs and their resistance. *Eur J Pharmacol.* 2014; 741C:156–70.

HIGHLIGHT 8

Nutrients, Herbals, and Phytochemicals: Do They Affect Cancer or Not?

Throughout this chapter, we discussed how large amounts of nutrients and phytochemicals have an impact upon biological processes related to disease incidence and progression. Perhaps the most significant relationship to disease, as well as the most debated, is the prevention of cancers at various sites. As of the most recent report provided by the Centers for Disease Control (CDC), cancer was the second leading cause of death in the United States, about 1% less than deaths due to heart disease. The rates for both were much higher than those for all other causes, 24.1% for heart disease and 23.3% for cancer. Obviously, we need to know whether nutrients and phytochemicals can make a difference. Although we know that some cancers have genetic origins, environment clearly is also important. Tobacco, diet, activity, and toxic materials all can influence cancer incidence and progression.

This Highlight attempts to deliver to the reader a contemporary understanding of the role of nutrients and phytochemicals in cancer incidence as debated by contemporary scientists knowledgeable in this area. Clear differences are present in their opinions, but the goal is to understand the facts as currently known.

Starting with an upbeat perspective, there seems to be some potential for clinical use of curcumin, according to early clinical studies. The best results appear in patients at risk for colorectal cancer and those that already have pancreatic cancer. Obstacles that face clinicians are the very poor absorption of dietary curcumin, so extremely high levels need to be used. Curcumin in conjunction with other drugs may also result in a better prognosis for women with breast cancer. Use of combined therapies could result in lower levels of curcumin being used in the treatment.

The use of complementary and alternative medicine (CAM) by cancer patients has gained much traction as cancer becomes a greater threat to more lives. Currently, it is estimated that 50% to 60% of cancer patients are using some form of CAM. Some of the alternatives people seek include genistein, resveratrol, milk thistle, and garlic. Other possible alternative therapies include polyphenols from green tea, sulforaphane from broccoli, isothiocyanates from cruciferous vegetables, lycopene from tomatoes, and gingerol from ginger. Of course, clinical trials are necessary to determine the levels of the phytonutrients needed for optimal anticancer activity, so much work is to be accomplished.

According to informed critics, valid results from trials of these materials are unlikely. In general, answers to these questions for phytochemicals or synthetic or extracted pharmaceuticals will be difficult to determine due to differences between individuals as well as the fact that responses to these materials over time may decline due to bodily adaptations. Lessons can be learned from existing pharmacological treatments. For instance, the commonly used drug for treating breast cancer, tamoxifen, will eventually stop working for some women as the cancer cells adapt to its use.

Suggested Readings

Patterson SL, Maresso KC, Hawk E. Cancer chemoprevention: Successes and failures. *Clin Chem.* 2013; 59:94–101.

Potter JD. The failure of cancer chemoprevention. *Carcinogenesis.* 2014; 35:974–82.

Thakur VS, Deb G, Babcock MA et al. Plant phytochemicals as epigenetic modulators: Role in cancer chemoprevention. *AAPS J.* 2014; 16:151–63.

Wang H, Khor TO, Shu L, et al. Plants against cancer: A review on natural phytochemicals in preventing and treating cancers and their druggability. *Anticancer Agents Med Chem.* 2012; 12:1281–305.

Wang J, Jiang Y.-F. Natural compounds as anticancer agents: experimental evidence. *WJEM.* 2012; 2:45–57.

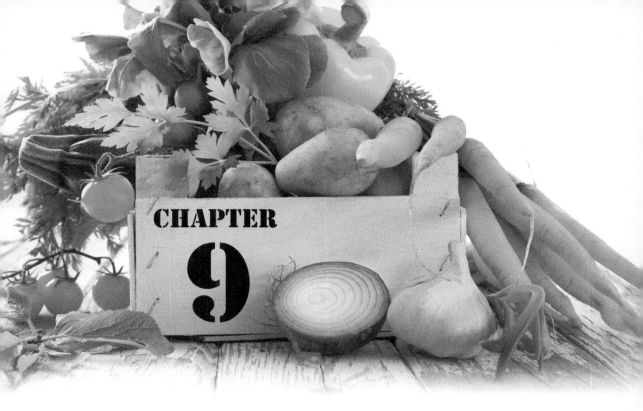

9

Nutrition and Fitness

This chapter is not organized similarly to the previous chapters on nutrients. It does not identify specific nutrients and their effects, but rather it is organized by the way that nutrient consumption affects the potential for individuals at different times relative to exercise. More specifically, it gives practical advice as to what nutrients and foods to consume prior to activity, during some activities, as well as after activity.

Nutrient Intake Prior to Activity

Nutrient intake prior to activity is probably the most important aspect for most people. The most significant nutrients to consume for most activities are carbohydrates and water, and the energy source most required during activity is glucose. Glucose use is mostly dependent upon the amount of glycogen, the glucose polymer found primarily in liver and muscle. Although the glycogen in muscle does provide glucose as a fuel source

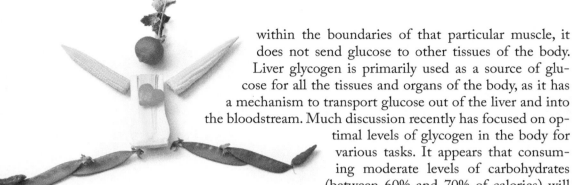

within the boundaries of that particular muscle, it does not send glucose to other tissues of the body. Liver glycogen is primarily used as a source of glucose for all the tissues and organs of the body, as it has a mechanism to transport glucose out of the liver and into the bloodstream. Much discussion recently has focused on optimal levels of glycogen in the body for various tasks. It appears that consuming moderate levels of carbohydrates (between 60% and 70% of calories) will provide adequate energy for most activities. If the activity is going to be particularly long or strenuous, then greater levels of con-

It is critical to consume adequate carbohydrates to maintain optimal fitness.

sumption become needed, usually about 70% to 80% of calories. For instance, when engaging in an endurance activity, a trained athlete may be able to perform an activity 50% longer when consuming a habitual higher-carbohydrate diet.

The major problem with not storing enough glycogen in the body is that the nervous system requires glucose; therefore, individuals experience dysfunctionality when they run out of glycogen or glucose. Interestingly, the highest percentage of total energy used from glucose occurs during the first twenty minutes or so of activity. Although glucose use continues, fat gradually displaces much of it. For this reason, we need to exercise beyond twenty minutes in order to start losing fat. Regular exercise encourages greater use of fat due to the muscles' better use of oxygen. Some experts have been encouraging the consumption of high-fat, low-carbohydrate diets for optimal performance. This strategy has met with extremely mixed results, with some trials showing that the high-fat diets result in only a third of the maximal performance time compared to high-carbohydrate diets. Other trials have also found greater fatigue in those performing an activity after habitual consumption of high-fat diets. In non-peer-reviewed literature, under conditions less than appropriately monitored, some reports suggest the benefits of high-fat diets prior to activity. Most sports nutritionists do not recommend a level lower than 20%, nor higher than 35%, as fat calories. This level is the same as would be advised for dietary intake for any adult.

Hydration is also significant, as the body uses water as a coolant through sweating. It is critical to be as hydrated as possible through optimal fluid intake prior to activity. It is recommended that from 1 to 3 cups of water be consumed prior to activity.

Nutrient Intake and Use during Activity

Nutrient intake and use during activity depend to a large extent on the activity. Although we have already mentioned that the body gradually adapts to using fat for energy, it continually uses between 30 and 60 grams per hour of glucose. Many people who exercise do so to increase their fitness, but many people are mostly concerned about losing or at least not gaining body fat.

Body fat that is lost due to energy use comes from internal sources as well as **subcutaneous** fat. Without question, those areas of the body typically provide the most fat for energy. The exception appears to be abdominal fat. Although the mechanism for its accumulation is favored by body metabolism, regrettably, the loss is not favored. As a result, the abdomen is an extremely resistant area and has defied numerous strategies to encourage loss of fat there. Some body fat is essential to provide cushioning and energy to the body, so it is not unanticipated that the body's metabolic activity will favor some fat retention.

Carbohydrates should certainly be consumed during prolonged activity. The carbohydrates should be in the form of the most absorbable form, glucose. The easiest way to get glucose into the body is to dissolve it in water and consume it throughout the activity. This enables the body to have a continuous supply of its preferred energy source for the central nervous system. Protein intake and its use during activity have been somewhat controversial. Although protein is not a major fuel for activity, many individuals exercise to increase their muscle mass, which requires protein storage. Ironically, muscle synthesis is actually reduced during activity. Only after the activity does the process of building more muscle begin.

As mentioned earlier, optimal hydration is important for best performance. Unfortunately, despite our excellent physiological systems to determine thirst, they usually only signal thirst to a vigorously active person after their body

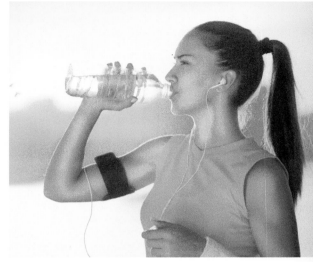

Subcutaneous: Below the skin.

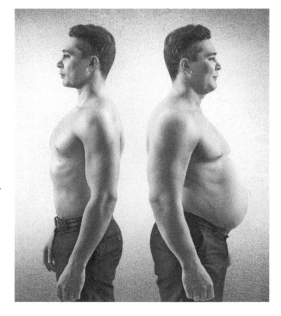

Abdominal fat accumulates and is difficult to remove without high levels of activity.

fluids are depleted. This reason makes it imperative to consume fluids during endurance activities, so that fluid depletion does not occur. Current recommendations are to consume one half to one cup of water every fifteen minutes. If dehydration does occur, it can result in disorientation and certainly suboptimal performance of an activity. In the worst-case scenario, heat stroke can occur, with great debilitation and possibly permanent consequences.

Many investigations have attempted to determine if micronutrients (vitamins and minerals) are required at higher levels for optimal performance. The suggested reasons include that many micronutrients encourage energy utilization, the transport of oxygen, water balance, muscle and nerve function, and the destruction of free radicals. A brief overview of some of the conclusions follows.

For nutrients involved in energy utilization, such as numerous water-soluble vitamins as well as minerals, there does not seem to be an advantage to consuming higher levels. Optimal use of energy should occur with the same intake suggested for other nutrients.

Electrolyte losses—sodium, potassium, and chloride—can be significant for those sweating profusely either due to prolonged activity or activity done when external temperatures are high. An imbalance of electrolytes can be injurious, particularly due to potassium losses. As mentioned, electrolytes are important for controlling water balance as well as being active in muscle contraction and nerve conduction. Consequently, fluids consumed during activity should include electrolytes, with an emphasis on potassium.

Potassium needs are high during exercise due to sweat losses – potassium from bananas can be helpful.

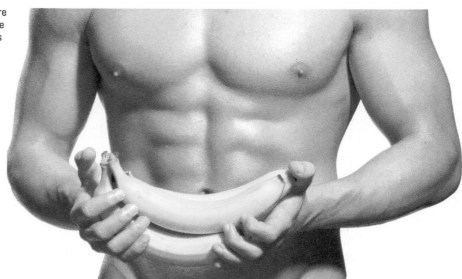

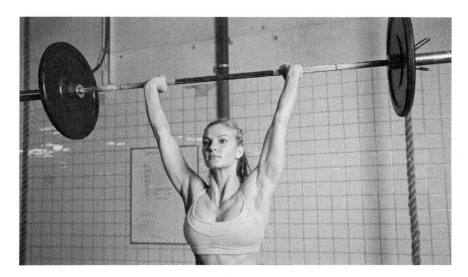

One mineral that has been studied thoroughly due to its significance in both oxygen transport and energy metabolism is iron. Studies have found that iron deficiency is common among young women and certainly among young female athletes. As a result, performance can be suboptimal. Although supplements may be necessary, iron status should be closely monitored. One striking finding has been *sports anemia*, a transient condition in which iron inadequacy may occur in athletes at the inception of an activity regimen but resolves soon afterward.

Numerous studies have looked at the possible impact of antioxidants upon performance. It has been postulated that a high level of antioxidants in the body prevents damage and encourages repair during activity. Although some people recommend vitamin E or vitamin C supplements to increase antioxidant capacity, these recommendations are premature as significant evidence exists that antioxidants may interfere with metabolic pathways that are beneficial. More research is needed in this area.

Nutrient Intake and Use after Activity

Nutrient intake and use after activity have been studied recently in order to understand what types of energy sources are most needed to replenish the losses of energy during activity as well as to increase muscle tissue. In addition, replenishment of body water has also been explored.

As for muscle, recent research suggests that high-quality protein is needed for rebuilding and increasing this tissue after activity. Although we covered earlier that most people were consuming far more protein than

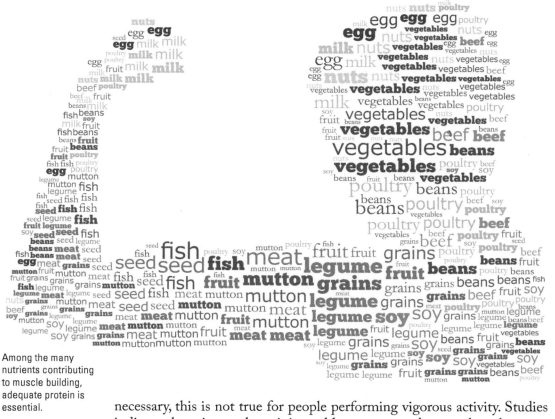

Among the many nutrients contributing to muscle building, adequate protein is essential.

necessary, this is not true for people performing vigorous activity. Studies indicate that vigorously training athletes may need somewhere between one and a half to two times the amount of protein required for more sedentary adults. This relationship appears to be true irrespective of gender. Fortunately, due to the dietary habits of most vigorously training men, their intake of protein is generally adequate for the amount needed. For vigorously training women, however, their intakes are often below what they actually should be consuming. Female athletes and other women performing vigorous activity should therefore consume additional dietary protein or supplementary sources.

There has been tremendous interest in fluid replenishment after activity, as we know that heavy sweating induced by exercise can result in water imbalance. In order to replenish the lost fluids, about 2 cups per pound of body weight lost during the activity should be adequate. We presume that the lost weight was primarily due to fluid. Research has demonstrated that not more than 2 cups of water should be consumed about every half hour until the required amount is consumed. This strategy appears to result in better water retention.

Carbohydrate intake after activity should also be included, as the body needs to replenish its stores of glycogen. If possible, intake should be spread out over the course of a day, but if the need to compete or be active occurs within the same day, the individual should consume the carbohydrates during the period that is available.

Suggested Readings

Beelen M, Burke LM, Gibala MJ, et al. Nutritional strategies to promote postexercise recovery. *Int J Sport Nutr Exerc Metab.* 2010; 20:515–32.

Burke LM, Hawley JA, Wong SH, et al. Carbohydrates for training and competition. *J Sports Sci.* 2011; 29 Suppl 1:S17–S27.

Genton L, Melzer K, Pichard C. Energy and macronutrient requirements for physical fitness in exercising subjects. *Clin Nutr.* 2010; 29:413–23.

Jeukendrup AE. Nutrition for endurance sports: Marathon, triathlon and road cycling. *J Sports Sci.* 2011; 29 Suppl 1:S91–S99.

Jeukendrup AE, Killer SC. The myths surrounding pre-exercise carbohydrate feeding. *Ann Nutr Metab.* 2010; 57(suppl 2):18–25.

Kraft JA, Green JM, Bishop PA, et al. The influence of hydration on anaerobic performance: A review. *Res Q Exerc Sport.* 2012; 83:282–92.

Phillips SM. Dietary protein requirements and adaptive advantages in athletes. *Br J Nutr.* 2012; Suppl 2:S158–S167.

HIGHLIGHT 9

Can Some Dietary and Nondietary Substances Enhance Performance?

For numerous decades, people have tried to determine whether some dietary and nondietary substances can enhance performance. Attempts at reaching a conclusion have taken shape as the result of individuals testing materials on themselves as well as scientists' controlled trials carried out on numerous individuals. Unfortunately, many substances have significant side effects or simply do not work.

On the other hand, some substances do appear to increase performance without serious side effects. In this Highlight, I attempt to separate out these categories in the hope that individuals can better ascertain appropriate use of certain substances.

Phytochemicals have been discussed, particularly as they may aid in either preventing or treating disease. Ginseng, in addition to its medical value, may also be valuable to prevent fatigue and therefore increase physical stamina and performance. Many of the naturally occurring phytochemical antioxidants may reduce muscle damage and fatigue. As stated previously, antioxidants must be consumed judiciously, as an excess may be injurious.

Some amino acids have also been suggested as performance enhancers. Arginine and ornithine are suspected to increase production of growth hormone, thus contributing to muscle growth. Aspartic acid salts have been reported to reduce fatigue. Branched amino acids, which include isoleucine, leucine, and valine, may reduce the levels of tryptophan entering the brain, thus reducing fatigue.

Several intermediary metabolites have been suggested to improve performance. For instance, bicarbonate may act as a buffer to lactic acid, which often builds up in the body and can cause fatigue. Carnitine has been explored as an aid to improve fatty acid use, based upon its known biochemical value in the use of fatty acids for energy. However, studies so far do not confirm carnitine's affect on fat during exercise. One of the more recent additions to the list of candidates is coenzyme Q_{10}, which is important for the ultimate extraction of energy from dietary materials. Some people have found that consuming creatine, a compound associated with muscle energy, may improve muscle stamina. Although promising, not enough research has been done to verify that increases in either beta-hydroxymethylbutyrate, a metabolite of leucine, or ribose, a 5-carbon sugar, improves muscle performance.

Some pharmacological substances have also been evaluated as performance enhancers. One of the most obvious choices is caffeine, commonly found in chocolate, numerous soft drinks, and of course, coffee and many teas. Although caffeine stimulates the central nervous system and likely enhances the availability of fatty acids, the potential for abuse is present. High intakes of caffeine and a similar substance known as *ma huang* can result in cardiac irregularities. In fact, the NCAA restricts use of caffeine for competition by athletes. Moreover, the FDA has banned sale of *ma huang*.

Alcohol, as ethanol, has many effects upon the body. Obviously, for many people it decreases their inhibitions, but unfortunately it also decreases their ability to respond to environmental conditions. Clearly, although some believe that alcohol enhances performance, it does the opposite.

Chromium picolinate, a salt of the mineral chromium, which is important for optimal use of glucose by the body, has been suggested to be a performance stimulant through building muscle and burning fat. Studies do not suggest that these enhancements are occurring.

Hormonal materials have long been suggested and used to enhance performance. The basic hormone is the androgen testosterone, which is responsible for virility and muscle strength and growth, particularly among men. Although testosterone itself has been demonstrated to have numerous serious side effects, such as abnormal growth of hair in women and inability to deal with stress in men, it is still being used. Of course, virtually all sports associations ban it, but it has found resurgence as a prescription drug to reduce the effects of aging in older males.

More commonly used are either herbal materials that stimulate the production of androgens by the body or materials similar to testosterone, like DHEA and androstenedione,

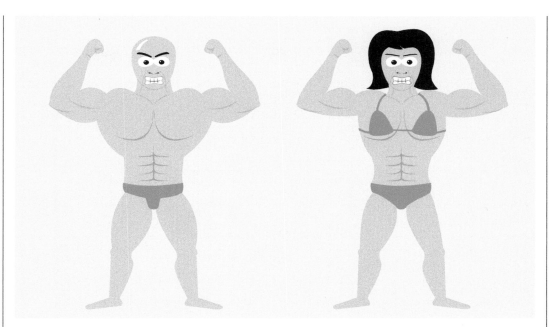

Steroids can have tremendous effects upon both men and women

made in the adrenal glands, which are used like testosterone to increase muscle. Although most sports associations also ban these testosterone-like hormones, some people who are not competing who wish to improve muscularity still use them.

Human growth hormone (HGH), produced by the pituitary gland, aids in the development of children and adolescents. Some individuals trying to gain a competitive edge have taken this hormone as adults. While it does seem to increase muscle mass, it also results in bone growth disruption. HGH is not a successful way to improve performance and is also banned by most sports associations.

Suggested Readings

Burke LM. Practical considerations for bicarbonate loading and sports performance. *Nestle Nutr Inst Workshop Ser.* 2013; 75:15–26.

Cherniack EP. Ergonenic dietary aids for the elderly. *Nutrition.* 2012; 28:225–9.

Peternelj TT, Coombes JS. Antioxidant supplementation during exercise training: beneficial or detrimental? *Sports Med.* 2011; 41:1043–69.

Rooney KB, Bryson JM, Digney AL, et al. Creatine supplementation affects glucose homeostasis but not insulin secretion in humans. *Ann Nutr Metab.* 2003; 47:11–15.

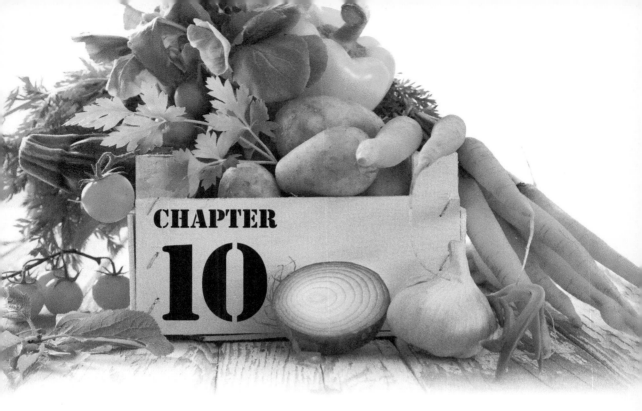

Globally Inadequate Nutrients

It is easy to be unaware of dietary issues that concern most of the developing and emerging world, as well as groups of individuals here in the United States. Two issues are of basic concern: the problem of providing already grown foodstuffs to individuals at risk and providing individuals with the skills to prepare or grow basic foods. I focused in the previous chapters on the needs and availability of nutrients and foods to most people in the United States, while in this chapter I address the needs versus the availability of nutrients and foods to developing and emerging nations as well as some groups of individuals in our own country. The emphasis is on several nutrients, including protein, calories, iron, and vitamin A—the major nutrients that seem to be inadequate for some of the groups identified earlier.

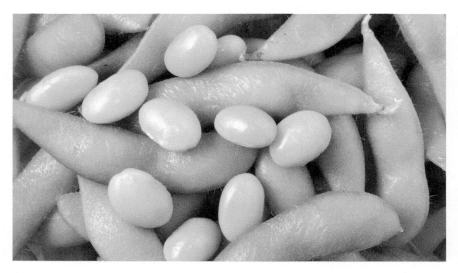

Soy products can be a valuable alternative to animal products as a protein food.

Protein and Calories

Protein and calories were discussed earlier in the context of nutrients that are often found in greater amounts than needed in the diets of many people in the United States. Ironically, protein is a major inadequate nutrient in many developing and emerging nations and to some extent for the poorer classes of individuals in the United States. The major reason for the inadequacy is that most people depend on protein from animal foods to ensure that they have the adequate essential amino acids as well as protein in general. When animal foods are not readily available, most people turn to plant materials to try and get enough of the essential amino acids and protein in general.

The ideal protein source, according to the United Nations' World Health Organization (WHO) and Food and Agricultural Organization (FAO), is similar to the protein in milk. In fact, we use this as a standard for evaluating protein sources. The basic calculation is to look at the individual amino acids in the protein being consumed compared to the ideal FAO/WHO amino acid profile. The amino acid that is the lowest compared to the standard is considered the limiting amino acid. The percentage of this amino acid compared to the standard is calculated. For instance, for many plant proteins, the limiting amino acids may be quite low. A figure of 20% would not be unusual, and we refer to that as the *amino acid score*. We multiply that number by the percentage of absorbability of that protein. For plant proteins, the absorbability would often be low; something like 80% may be the amount that the digestive system can absorb. If we multiply these two percentages together, we get a score called the Protein

Digestion Corrected Amino Acid Score (PDCAAS). In the case we are using, the corrected score would be 16%, which translates to an inadequate amount of essential amino acids provided to the individual. Often, the total amount of amino acids is also low, contributing to protein inadequacy.

Fortunately, many individuals have alternatives to being protein inadequate. For instance, vegans—strict vegetarians who do not eat animal products—often combine sources of protein that complement each other, providing a total amino acid amount that will have high percentages of all of the essential amino acids. Of course, they still need to be sure that they are getting sufficient protein from these sources. Another alternative is to consume plant proteins that already have a high content of all of the essential amino acids, similar to animal proteins. At this time the only common protein sources that could be employed for this purpose are soy and quinoa. There has also been a recent cultivation of quality protein maize (QPM), particularly in Sub-Saharan Africa. As we evaluate other plant materials, perhaps additional plant proteins may be found to be complete or can be modified.

Protein and calorie malnutrition persists as a problem in developing and emerging nations.

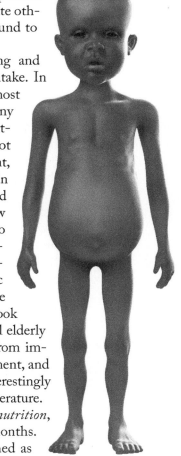

The problem of protein malnutrition in many developing and emerging nations is also complicated by inadequate energy intake. In fact, distinguishing between the two is very difficult, since they most commonly occur together. Inadequate calorie intake has many causes, but the most common are simply that food is not transported to individuals, they cannot afford to purchase it, or they cannot grow it due to inadequate environmental resources. In any event, we find that young children typically suffer the most, as they are in an intense developmental phase and need sufficient essential and nonessential amino acids to ensure that they develop and grow appropriately. Since adults have already developed and grown to their capacity, the major issue for them is a reduced immune system. Two conditions that can develop in small children are marasmus and kwashiorkor. *Marasmus* can be described as chronic protein and energy malnutrition in small children. In general, the condition occurs between 6 and 18 months of age. The children look emaciated, their skin shrivels, and they appear to look like small elderly people. In addition to their appearance, they generally suffer from impaired growth, wasting of muscles, and impaired brain development, and have difficulties in their ability to digest and absorb food. Interestingly they also have difficulties in maintaining an adequate body temperature.

Kwashiorkor, also known as *acute protein and energy malnutrition*, generally develops rapidly in children between 18 and 24 months. Ironically, these children may appear to be adequately nourished as

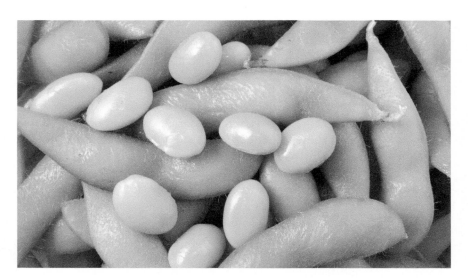

Soy is an excellent substitute for animal protein.

they generally have edema. This makes them appear robust, as the water that accumulates can easily be mistaken for fat accumulation. Internally, however, these children have fatty liver, inflammation, and immune system impairment. If observed closely, they also have external appearances indicative of malnourishment, including changes to their skin and hair texture.

In reality, differentiating between these two types of protein and calorie malnutrition is often difficult, and many times there is a mix of the two, with edema as well as degeneration associated with both types of protein and calorie inadequacy. Whether a child or adult is afflicted with this malnutrition, the ultimate consequences seem similar. Typically, there are systemic infections due to protein inadequacies that cannot sustain the immune system. In addition, diarrhea is extremely common due to the inability of the digestive system to digest foods and absorb nutrients and water. The heart, perhaps the most important muscle in the body, is unable to sustain its activity, and heart failure often occurs. All of these conditions contribute to the high mortality rate associated with protein and calorie malnutrition globally. If aid arrives in time, rehydration is extremely critical, followed by the addition of calories and protein to the diet, although this must be done gradually.

Iron

Iron deficiency is a major global health issue. Although we have some concerns about specific population groups in the United States, our food supply is supplemented with iron and ample supplements are available. In developing and emerging nations, iron intake is inadequate due to the types of food consumed; neither food supplementation with iron nor supplements are available to improve iron status. You may recall that iron deficiency was discussed previously in highlighting nutrients often inadequate in diets in the United States. Indeed, serious deficiency effects relate to the immune system and development, but most people here are diagnosed and provided with supplements.

Iron inadequacy persists as a serious health problem in many places in the world. As stated previously, the form of iron that is most bioavailable is heme iron, present in animal foods, but many places in the world have a shortage of animal foods. Although there is iron in plant materials, the amount that the body can absorb is comparatively low. In addition there are interfering factors in plant foods, like phytic acid, commonly found in wheat and soy. An additional problem not generally encountered domestically is the presence of parasites in the body that sequester the iron, rendering it unavailable. As a result of these issues, iron inadequacy is the most common nutrient deficiency globally. In particular, the deficiency is most common in women during their reproductive years, especially during pregnancy. It is also quite common in infants, young children, and adolescents.

The consequences of iron deficiency are severe, with a diminished ability to use energy-yielding nutrients due to the lack of oxygen transport to tissues and the iron-containing substances that extract energy. As a result, individuals have a reduced capacity for both mental and physical activity and generally suffer from motivational issues. Numerous international agencies are making efforts to improve iron nutriture globally, but the basic problems of inadequate animal products and the low absorption from plant products and supplements are serious hindrances. Efforts have primarily focused on various methods of providing supplements to the target individuals identified earlier. The current strategies include increasing the iron in food crops, providing iron supplements through staples such as milk and cereal, and the use of a proprietary product known as Sprinkles, which people can literally sprinkle on any foodstuff. The formulations vary, and besides iron, numerous other nutrients are being used.

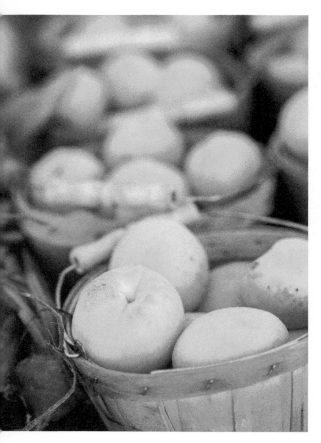

Despite the global abundance of foods containing carotenoids, vitamin A deficiency remains a serious problem.

Vitamin A

Vitamin A deficiency is a problem for many developing and emerging nations. In particular, East Asia, Central and South America, and Sub-Saharan Africa have been places where vitamin A deficiency is rampant. As discussed, the best sources of vitamin A other than animal liver are colorful fruits and vegetables, like carrots, sweet potatoes, and green vegetables. Although the carotenoids, the precursors of vitamin A, are generally orange or yellow, the green chlorophyll masks the color in many green vegetables.

Vitamin A deficiency can result in serious problems for the young and adult alike. Since the body requires vitamin A for the integrity of skin and mucus membranes, a deficiency leads to degeneration of the digestive system, trachea, and urinary tract. Also, the skin becomes hardened in a process called *keratinization*. This is due to overproduction of a protein called *keratin*, which is normally produced at low levels when vitamin A is adequate. Most individuals with vitamin A deficiency also experience a decrease in their immune response to disease. In fact, in countries where vitamin A deficiency is common, measles is a serious threat to survival. Other diseases are also worsened by the weak immune system, including malaria, tuberculosis, and AIDS. In addition, vitamin A is essential for both night vision as well as maintaining the integrity of the eye itself. Typically, children with inadequate intake of vitamin A go blind due to the degeneration of their eyes and also experience other forms of malnutrition due to damage to their digestive system. In addition, bone remodeling, a process critical to child development, is altered. Adults experience similar symptoms as children, but in addition they also lose their ability to reproduce. In the case of men, sperm are not produced, and in women, the fertilized egg cannot attach to the uterine wall. In summary, vitamin A deficiency is associated with greater risk of infectious disease, blindness, infertility in adults, and ultimately death.

Efforts to eradicate vitamin A deficiency globally have not yet proven successful, although progress has been made. The key strategy has been to place a vitamin A–containing oil on people's tongues and have them

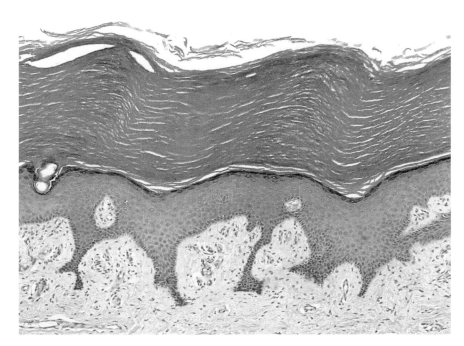

Keratinization due to vitamin A deficiency results in a rough, hardened skin.

swallow it. Fortunately, vitamin A is easily stored by the liver, so this process does not need to be repeated very often, perhaps several times a year. In addition, the crops in these regions are often filled with vitamin A precursors or carotenoids. The problem has been getting the people in the region to actually consume these crops. Many cultures value animal foods and do not consider plant foods of much value. In addition, they can sell these crops at the marketplace and subsist on the money earned. The problem of vitamin A inadequacy is not easy to solve, as the cultural obstacles are enormous.

Suggested Readings

Godfrey HC, Beddington JR, Crute IR, et al. Food security: The challenge of feeding 9 billion people. *Science.* 2010; 327:812–8.

Milman N. Anemia—still a major health problem in many parts of the world. *Ann Hematol.* 2011; 90:368–77.

Nuss ET, Tanumihardjo SA. Quality protein maize for Africa: Closing the protein inadequacy gap in vulnerable populations. *Adv Nutr.* 2011; 2:217–24.

Sommer A, Vyas KS. A global clinical view on vitamin A and carotenoids. *Am J Clin Nutr.* 2012; 96:1204S–1206S.

HIGHLIGHT 10

Genetically Engineered Crops as a Solution to Food and Nutrient Inadequacy?

As chapter 10 describes, serious global problems relate to obtaining adequate food and nutrients. One solution explored by scientists for several decades has been to genetically modify particular crops, either to make them more resistant to pests, increase their nutrient content, or increase their yield. Although natural selection and crop breeding have been around for thousands of years, the time taken to breed a crop with desirable characteristics can be extremely long. Genetic engineering involves the insertion of a gene or genes from other species into the genome of a particular plant and then propagating it so that it has the selected traits. This process is relatively fast in comparison. The crops are referred to as genetically modified organisms (GMOs). Some of the initial work involved adding to corn a gene for pest resistance. This proprietary process has led to greater yields of corn with less use of pesticide. Other scientists have produced soybeans that are able to produce better yields. Of course, this approach solves some of the problems inherent in areas that cannot produce enough food to ensure that all of the local residents get adequate protein and calories, particularly since soybeans are an excellent source of quality protein.

Another significant use of genetically modified crops has been to try and use genetic engineering to improve crops' nutrient content. This approach has been tested in at least two crops, one that was successful and the other not very successful from a consumer perspective. The case of increasing the vitamin A precursor beta-carotene in tomatoes was technically successful. Unfortunately, the public expects tomatoes to be red, but these were yellow-orange. Typically tomatoes produce a high level of lycopene, which gives them their red color. Lycopene may have some valuable health effects in preventing prostate cancer, but it is not a precursor for vitamin A. Although beta-carotene is the best plant source as a precursor to vitamin A, it is yellow-orange. Consumers would not accept this color change, so the experiment was a failure. Great success, though, has come for "golden rice," which has a gene inserted in the rice genome to increase the production of beta-carotene. Normally rice is not a good source of vitamin A, so this is a good example of improving the nutrient content of a globally common food. Consumer acceptability has been excellent, which will undoubtedly lead to fewer cases of vitamin A deficiency around the world.

Genetic engineering of food crops may come with a price. Although most domestic and international agencies have encouraged its use, some have advocated caution. Although the naysayers are extremely opposed to the use of GMOs, virtually all of their rhetoric has been either blatantly false, exaggerated, or based upon a few case studies. Some issues should be watched with caution include the potential for allergens being produced in the crops, "drifting" of the GMOs, and the development of an attitude aversive to crop rotation. Let's look at each of these potential issues and consider the possible consequences as well as the possible solutions.

First, many individuals have been concerned about the production of allergens in the crops. If this was to occur at all, it would not likely be due directly to the inserted gene. The gene will produce whatever protein it was intended to produce, but it is unlikely that any of these are common allergens. The consequences of altering the metabolism in the plant, however, could conceivably result in gene products that may be allergens. To date, we are unaware of this happening, but it is a possibility. The best defense against this possibility is to test the entire food being produced as a genetically modified crop for allergens. Although laborious, this process would solve the problem.

Second, the drifting of genetically modified crops from established locations to neighboring farms is a real problem and does have consequences. If the modified crop is more resistant to disease, then it will likely invade the neighboring crops that have not been modified. Many farmers pride themselves on their heirloom crops, and the corruption of these crops by the genetically modified plants can result in their crops no longer being traditional. This effect could cause a great economic as well as cultural loss. On the other hand, some neighboring farmers have made use of the drifting of the genetically modified crops to use the resultant seeds to produce heartier crops on their land. The courts have found that if the drifted crops are used unintentionally, then nothing is wrong with the benefit conferred to the neighboring farmers. If, however, as in some instances, they have intentionally benefited by harvesting the seeds and not paid the required royalties to the company that created the modified crop, then they are criminally negligent. Ways to prevent this occurrence include having a buffer zone that would serve as a barrier to the transfer of the crops with a modified genome to the neighboring farms.

Crop rotation, or the planting of diverse crops on the same soil in alternating years, has been a staple of farming for many years. The benefits that result are mostly related to the nutritional value of the soil, as different crops use different nutrients and continuous planting of the same crop can easily result in soil depletion. The incentive to keep planting the same genetically modified crop is obvious in that the genetically modified crop provides better yields. Therefore, the farmer is reticent to rotate crops. This problem needs to be fixed, and as yet there is no solution.

For those averse to genetically modified crops, one of the solutions they propose is to modify the pests instead. In this case, the pests are modified in such a way that they would feed or reproduce on some other plant, like a weed, rather than the crop of value. There may be other alternatives, but for now, in order to better feed the world's populations, GMOs seem to be a valuable strategy.

[Author's note: I would like to acknowledge the contribution of Sonia Shafner, who kindly supplied me with her undergraduate thesis titled "Genetically Engineered Crops: Proceed with Caution," which was submitted in partial fulfillment for her bachelor's degree in biology from the S. Daniel Abraham Honors Program at Stern College for Women in 2014. Many of the concepts in this Highlight drew heavily from her research into this topic.]

Suggested Readings

Dona A, Arvanitoyannis IS. Health risks of genetically modified foods. *Critical Rev in Food Sci and Nutrition.* 2009; 49:164-75.

Jones DL, Cross P, Withers PJA, et al. Nutrient stripping: The global disparity between food security and soil nutrient stocks. *J Appl Ecol.* 2013; 50:851–62.

Tang, G, Qin J, Dolnikowski GG, et al. Golden rice is an effective source of vitamin A. *Am J Clin Nutr.* 2009; 89:1776–83.

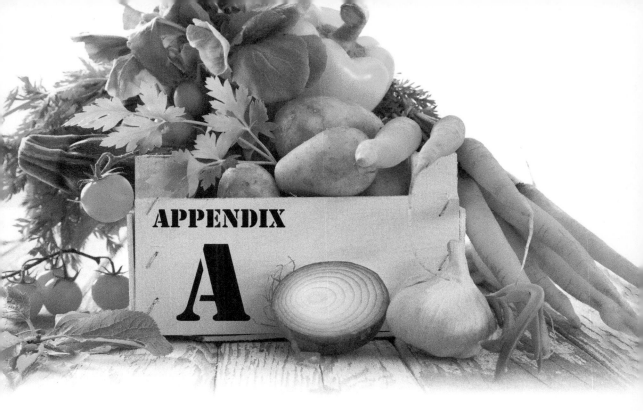

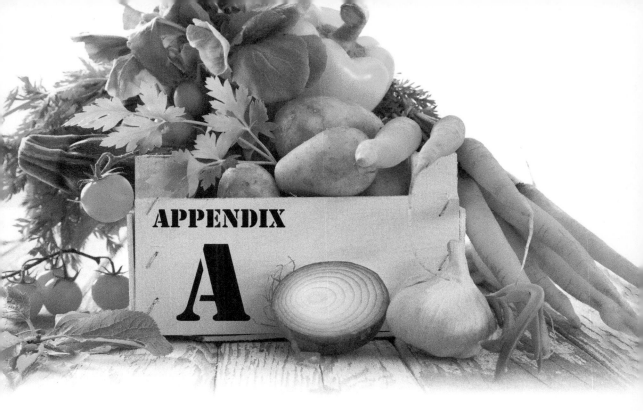 APPENDIX

A

Useful Websites and Links

The government and private sector each maintain a variety of websites that are particularly useful to support either selected chapters or a variety of chapters in the text as noted.

www.iom.edu
Summaries of the reports issued by the Food and Nutrition Board of the Institute of Medicine. The material here is relevant throughout the textbook.

www.usda.gov
Good information on how to use the dietary guidelines issued by the U.S. Department of Agriculture. In particular, *www.cnpp.usda.gov* provides a broad array of material concerning the function of the Center

for Nutrition Policy and Promotion with links to the Dietary Reference Intakes. This site is mostly useful when studying chapters 1 and 2 of the text. The material at *www.cnpp.usda.gov/healthyeatingindex* supplements Highlight 2 extremely well.

www.choosemyplate.gov
Extremely useful site maintained by the Department of Agriculture to help understand the role of MyPlate in determining good nutritional intake. This site is mostly relevant to chapter 2.

www.cdc.gov
The Centers for Disease Control website is very helpful in understanding the risks of disease from improper nutrition, including contaminants in food. Although in general it is most relevant to chapters 1 and 10, *www.cdc.gov/nutrition/index.html* is particularly relevant to areas like fitness, obesity, and exercise and is useful to further your understanding of chapters 7 and 9. In addition, this site also has a section on the NHANES dietary survey discussed in Highlight 1: *www.cdc.gov/nchs/nhanes.htm*.

www.fda.gov
This website, maintained by the Food and Drug Administration, would be particularly significant for finding additional information related to Highlights 7, 8 and 9.

www.letsmove.gov
This website is sponsored by an interdisciplinary group of government agencies to try and discourage childhood obesity and obesity in general. Currently led by Michelle Obama, the goal is to virtually eliminate childhood obesity by 2030. In particular, this site would provide useful information that primarily relates to chapter 7 and Highlight 7.

www.eatright.org
This website is sponsored by the Academy of Nutrition and Dietetics, the professional society that enables dietitians to become registered and sets the credentials for the registration process. As such, it also provides numerous interesting articles and material about a variety of disorders that dietary inadequacy and excess cause. It would be useful to further understanding of chapters 3–8, the chapters dedicated to nutrient needs.

www.hhs.gov
This website is maintained by the Health and Human Services division of the U.S. government. Although many aspects are of a more general health interest, a very useful component is www.foodsafety.gov, which is very useful in understanding more about the safety of our food supply. It is a good supplement for Appendix E.

www.nutrition.org
Sponsored by the American Society of Nutrition, a large group of nutrition professionals, this site provides useful information about many nutrients and offers numerous links to nutrition-related subjects. It should be useful as a supplement to most of this book, but in particular chapters 3–8.

www.heart.org
Sponsored by the American Heart Association, this website is devoted to many issues that promote awareness of or prevent heart disease. Since we discuss many aspects of diet that may affect cardiac performance, particularly those sections on fat intake, this site would be valuable for people who are interested in the discussion of fats in chapters 3 and 7.

www.health.gov
Sponsored by the U.S. Department of Health and Human Services, this website is devoted to providing recommendations for essential nutrients and for exercise. Links to the DRIs can be found at *www.dietaryguidelines. gov.* This site would be particularly useful as a supplement to chapter 9.

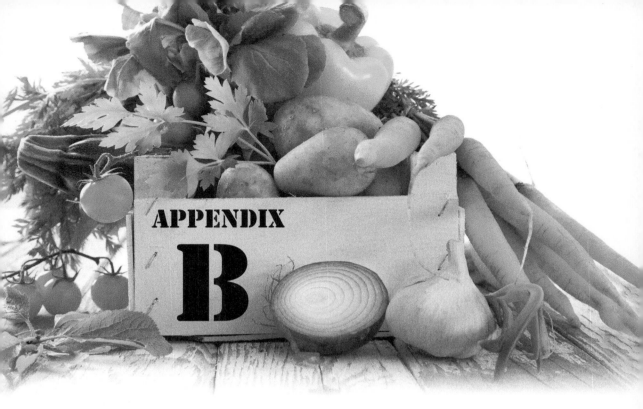

Digestion and Absorption

Although we typically discuss these two processes together, they are separate physiological actions. As such, we need to delineate where one process ends and the next begins, as together they are necessary for transporting individual nutrients to our circulatory system. It is also important to know where problems can occur in these processes, preventing us from either deriving all the benefits from our food or causing illness.

The *digestive system* can be divided into two components: the digestive tract and the accessory organs that provide various secretions to encourage digestion in the digestive tract. The digestive tract begins with the oral cavity (the mouth), passes to the esophagus, and then is followed by the stomach, small intestine, and finally the large intestine (usually referred to as the colon). Although the walls of these organs provide some secretions, the accessory organs—such as the salivary glands, the pancreas, the liver, and the gall bladder—also contribute secretions.

Of course, when we eat, food enters through our oral cavity. In addition to the obvious chewing of food, the mouth is the first place we encounter secretions, in this case coming from our salivary glands. At least three different types of salivary glands surround our mouths, and their secretions serve very useful purposes. Among them are the entry of water used for moistening the dry foods we consume to enable us to chew and swallow them. Saliva also contains numerous antimicrobial substances that reduce the population of microbes causing tooth decay and also contribute to disease prevention by killing many of these microbes before they proceed to the rest of the digestive system. Failure of the salivary glands to produce adequate saliva often leads to accelerated tooth decay and difficulty in chewing and swallowing dry foods. This condition often occurs after radiation therapy or simply due to the aging process. Artificial lubricants similar to saliva can be consumed to prevent these problems.

The mouth is connected to the esophagus by the pharynx, which is a small tube in the back of our mouths. The most significant problem that can occur here is due to swallowing and talking at the same time. The trachea, our breathing tube, also opens here. When we talk, a small flap of skin known as the epiglottis is opened so that we can use our vocal cords to speak. When we swallow, this flap closes to allow the food to enter our esophagus. Choking is mostly the result of trying to do both at the same time, with the consequences being that we aspirate food into our trachea. If the food gets stuck here, we cannot breathe, which can be life-threatening. If we aspirate the food more deeply, it often lodges in our respiratory tract and can cause disease, including pneumonia.

Our esophagus is the first place in the digestive tract where food begins to progress passively, as opposed to our oral cavity, which requires us to actively use muscles to swallow our food. The chewed food, which we refer to as bolus, is pushed through by a wavelike motion called peristalsis. These waves are controlled by the nervous system and do not require our participation. The esophagus, although not absolutely required for life, does seem to serve a useful purpose as a barrier between the stomach and the mouth. At the end of the esophagus is a muscle referred to as the cardiac sphincter, a valve that generally opens only to allow food to pass into the stomach. It can, however, allow food to pass back from the stomach, which generally does not occur unless sufficient pressure is present to push the valve in this direction. Situations that can cause this occurrence include vomiting, pregnancy, and indigestion. Most times, the results are temporary and not very serious or prolonged. We often refer to the return of stomach contents as "heartburn," due to the fact that the cardiac sphincter at the bottom of the esophagus is very near the heart. Due to the acidity of the stomach contents, we feel pain near our heart, even though it has nothing to do with our hearts. Many emergency room trips result in the diagnosis of heartburn, but unfortunately other individuals presume they have heartburn and do not go to the emergency room and may die due to a heart attack. Gastroesophageal reflux disorder (GERD) results from persistent heartburn that eventually erodes the esophagus. It is often worsened by consumption of chocolate, alcohol, and high-fat foods, as well as smoking. Some people believe that this constant irritation may encourage cancer of the esophagus. In any event it can be very painful and often results in persistent coughing and nausea.

Although the stomach can actually be divided into four main regions, the bottom of it, known as the antrum, results in the greatest contribution to digestion. In the antrum, the food is ground and mixed with stomach secretions, chiefly hydrochloric acid secreted by the stomach walls. Although digestion in the stomach is minimal, it focuses upon the initial breakdown of protein. While hydrochloric acid serves to "denature" or alter protein from its natural structure, one protease enzyme, pepsin, begins the process of removing amino acids from the various protein chains found in our food. Although some mixture of foods takes place throughout the stomach due to the several types of muscles in the walls, the major peristaltic activity occurs in the antrum. This peristalsis enables the food, which we now refer to as "chyme," to pass through another sphincter at the bottom of the stomach. This valve almost always functions to allow passage of digestive material only toward the small intestine and is referred to as the pyloric sphincter. Although small intestinal materials can pass back to the stomach, it is an unusual occurrence and is cause for medical intervention, as it is likely caused by blockage of the small intestine. The small intestine is filled with microorganisms and is an environment that can accommodate them, while the stomach is not a place where high levels of microorganisms can exist without negative consequences.

A much too common disorder of the gastrointestinal tract is an ulcer, which can occur in the bottom of the stomach or at the top of the small intestine. Theories of its occurrence and prevention were originally based upon dietary intake. We now know that there are probably three critical factors that cause the erosion of the lining of the gastrointestinal tract in these places: excess hydrochloric acid secretion, overuse of nonsteroidal anti-inflammatory drugs (NSAIDs, like aspirin and Advil), and the presence of the bacteria known as H. pylori. H. pylori appears to increase with age and may explain why more cases of ulcer occur in older individuals. Ulcers are painful and, if not reversed by medical treatment, can result in erosion severe enough to cause life-threatening bleeding of the gastrointestinal walls.

The small and large intestine together complete the passageway of food through the gastrointestinal tract. Peristalsis is very significant in making sure that our food passes through these areas. Later in this appendix we discuss the significance of the absorption of nutrients in both of these organs, but for now our attention focuses on the digestive processes. As in the stomach, some secretions act to break down the components of chyme to smaller molecules that can be absorbed. In addition to these secretions, some come from the accessory organs—the pancreas and the gall bladder—which also facilitate digestion. The pancreas produces numerous enzymes that break down protein, carbohydrate, and fat. The exception is fiber, which enzymes produced by the human body cannot break down. The gall bladder, although it does not produce enzymes, does secrete bile, which the body uses to solubilize fat so that the pancreatic enzymes can break it down. Bile is not actually produced by the gall bladder but is made by the liver. The liver secretes the bile into the gall bladder, where it is stored until the body needs it to enable the digestion of fat. As a result of the secretions in the small intestine, proteins are broken down into amino acids; starch is broken down into glucose; and fats are broken down into fatty acids, glycerol, and monoacylglycerol—all of which the small intestine can absorb.

Several major obstacles to the digestive process can occur in the small intestine. Perhaps the most serious is the lack of pancreatic enzymes, which could be caused by disease or age. The only solution is to provide these enzymes in a capsule that opens up in the small intestine and functions like those that the pancreas would have secreted. The other obstacle is the lack of bile, due usually to a dysfunctional gall bladder or blockage of the duct leading from the gall bladder into the small intestine, which results in a lack of fat digestion. After removing the gall bladder, most surgeons simply attach the original duct from the liver to the small intestine. The positive side of this process is that bile is available to help solubilize the fat. The negative side is that the bile constantly drips into the small intestine, greatly increasing the risk of colon cancer, as the bile's metabolites are cancer-causing.

The material that enters the colon is composed of water, fiber, and other materials from food that the small intestine could not digest or absorb adequately. The colon is able to absorb water and electrolytes like sodium and chloride. The large number of microorganisms are also able to break down many fibers into short-chain fatty acids like butyric and propionic acid.

Several other issues can commonly arise related to the digestive tract. One of the most common is appendicitis. This disorder occurs as a result of food and bacteria entering a small pouch that is located very close to where the colon connects to the small intestine. When the bacteria start to grow, an infection results, causing great pain. The only cure is to have the appendix removed, because if the condition is allowed to progress, the appendix can burst and result in systemic infection.

The *absorptive system* enables our bodies to use the products of digestion and those nutrients that do not require digestion by allowing absorption of these materials across the cells of the gastrointestinal tract and into the circulatory system. Although many drugs and other small molecules may be absorbed through the walls of the stomach, it is believed that absorption of nutrients primarily occurs in the small intestine. The small intestine is uniquely formed in a way that optimizes the transfer of nutrients across its walls and into the circulatory system. Numerous enterocytes (cells of absorption) line the many folds of the small intestinal lining. These enterocytes transport both the fatty and the water-soluble materials that are traveling through the small intestine. These cells are in proximity to both circulatory systems. One, known as the lymphatic system, picks up fatty materials and brings them to the body. The types of materials it transports include the fats and the fat-soluble vitamins like vitamins A, D, E, and K. The other circulatory system, known as the arterio-venous system, picks up the amino acids from protein digestion; sugars; the water-soluble vitamins like thiamin, niacin, riboflavin, folate, and vitamin B_{12}; and minerals. Some absorption occurs in the large intestine, but it appears to be limited to water, electrolytes, and fiber fermentation products like butyric and propionic acid.

Numerous problems can occur with respect to optimal absorption. One of the key issues is diarrhea. If food passes too quickly through the small and large intestine, then neither digestion nor absorption will occur optimally because there is not enough time for the food to be in proximity to the enzymes, cells, and so on. Consequently, nutrients can't be optimally absorbed into the body, nor can water be reabsorbed for body use. Perhaps one of the most common problems that is still not satisfactorily understood is irritable bowel syndrome (IBS). In this fairly common condition, it is believed that the nervous system, which regulates the passage of food through the small and large intestines, is not operating properly. Some clinicians and researchers believe that some of the problem may be due to the type of bacteria inhabiting the colon. In an effort to alleviate the symptoms of IBS, which can range from diarrhea to constipation, many clinicians recommend the consumption of either pre- or probiotics. Prebiotics are food materials that encourage the growth of healthy bacteria in the colon. Probiotics are bacteria that are consumed in large enough quantities to repopulate the colon of IBS suffers with bacteria that are more conducive to a healthy colon. Probiotics are also thought to reduce colonization by pathogenic bacteria, promote excretion of toxic substances and increase fecal bulk.

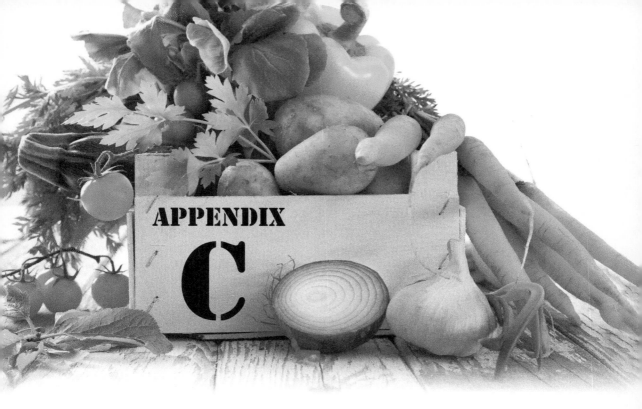

Nonnutritive Dietary Components

Much discussion concerns the various materials that are added to our food for flavor, texture, and other sensory purposes. A full discussion of all of these materials would take a full semester and a lot more space than an appendix provides. This appendix is devoted only to a small group of additives, as these are the ones most significant to a nutrition course, as opposed to a course in food science. Consequently, the three areas of discussion are sugar substitutes, fat substitutes, and artificial fibers.

Sugar substitutes, or *nonnutritive sweeteners*, were developed for several reasons. One reason is that that diabetics generally need to curtail their intake of sugar to prevent glucose and insulin surges. Another reason is that since they are noncaloric, an individual who is trying to reduce caloric intake but still wants to consume sweet foods ingests fewer calories from their sweetened foods when nonnutritive sweeteners are substituted for sugars.

Third, these sweeteners are not used by the bacteria in the mouth for growth, so their substitution for sugars decreases the development of dental caries. The two major types of sugar substitutes are artificial and herbal sweeteners.

Several different artificial sweeteners are commonly used. Perhaps the most controversial substitute is *aspartame*, commonly marketed as NutraSweet. Chemically, it comprises two amino acids linked together: phenylalanine and aspartic acid. Technically, it provides the same calories as either sugar or protein, but the amount required to sweeten beverages and other foodstuffs is so small that its contribution to total calories consumed is very small. In fact, aspartame is about 200 times sweeter than a similar quantity of sucrose or table sugar. Although safe for most people, some individuals are born with an inherited disorder called *phenylketonuria*. These individuals cannot metabolize excess phenylalanine and must restrict their intake of this amino acid. Because of this problem, a warning label must appear on all products using this artificial sweetener so that individuals with this disorder can make an informed decision. Serious consequences can develop for those individuals who consume excess levels of aspartame, including disturbances to the nervous system.

Saccharin is another commonly used sugar substitute in the United States. Due to its chemical structure, it does not provide any caloric value but does provide a high level of sweetness, actually about double the amount of aspartame.

Cyclamates were very popular some time ago in the United States until they were banned. Although still available in Canada, they are not yet available again in the United States, even though they have been demonstrated to be safe at the level typically consumed. Cyclamates, like saccharin, are completely nonnutritive but have a considerably lower capacity to sweeten beverages and foods.

Other alternative sweeteners being commercially used include Acesulfame K and Sucralose, which also provide great levels of sweetening capacity without any caloric value. You may notice many products that use these newer materials as well.

Stevia is the only herbal sweetener available in the United States. Marketed as Truvia, South Americans have long used stevia to sweeten beverages. It is a glycoside derived from the leaves of a particular plant. As a consequence it does not have caloric value but does have a very high sweetening value compared to table sugar. Since it is on the FDA's GRAS (generally recognized as safe) list of materials that can be added to food and beverages, stevia is presumed to be safe until otherwise proven differently.

Fat substitutes are becoming more common in food production, as we become more concerned about the high caloric value of fat and also as we have become more aware of many individuals' limitations for fat digestion and absorption, primarily due to the aging process. The industry has responded to these needs with fat, protein, and carbohydrate derivatives that simulate the texture of fat in foods without the calories or need to digest fat.

Although the industry uses derivatives of all these macronutrients for a variety of purposes, including texture and emulsification, olestra is by far the most common ingredient used as a fat replacement, primarily in chips and crackers. It lacks the undesirable characteristics of fat, such as caloric value, digestive challenges, and negative health consequences associated with heart disease and specific types of cancer, because it is not a fat. In fact, it cannot be digested; although there are fatty acids in it, they are attached to a sucrose (table sugar) molecule. The human digestive system does not have the capacity to break down these bonds, so the olestra molecule has no caloric value. Unfortunately, olestra does bind to the various fat-soluble vitamins (A, D, E, and K), and as a result they can be more readily lost from the digestive tract. If used in a product, the olestra must be fortified with these vitamins to discourage the molecule from binding to the vitamins that are coming naturally from other components of the diet.

Fiber substitutes have become more common as we realize that fiber is important to our health and that most of us do not consume enough of it. The food industry has responded with *functional fiber*, a term that describes materials that are either isolated, extracted, or manufactured and can be shown to have value as a fibrous material in the human diet. Many functional fibers are present in plants that are not generally edible by humans and are extracted for use in foods that we do eat. For example, cellulose, pectin, lignin, gums, beta-glucans, fructans, and resistant starches are all dietary fibers. In other words, they are part of the fiber consumption we already have from consuming the plant materials that are a normal part of our diet. Other materials being used in processed foods are also not normal constituents of our fiber intake but have properties that are similar to those substances. Included in this group are chitan and chitosan, polydextrose and polyols, psyllium, and resistant dextrins. Other than chitan and chitosan, which are derived from the shells of water-inhabiting animals, the rest are either extracts from plants we do not consume or are products of the food industry. Many fiber substitutes are still undergoing extensive testing to demonstrate their health value in the human diet. Some are being used in countries outside of the United States, while others are being used here. Hopefully, future research can determine whether these functional fibers are indeed valuable additives to our diet.

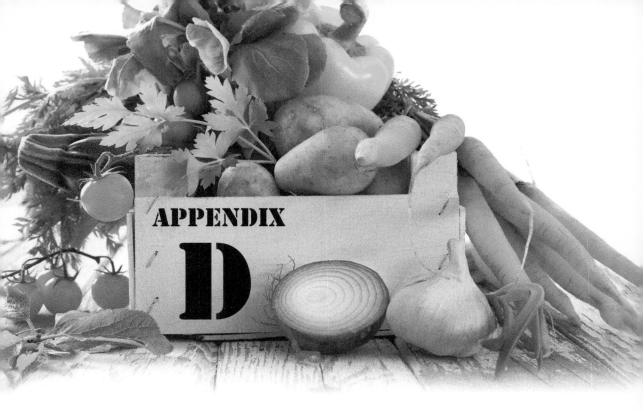

Cells, Genetics, and Protein Synthesis

The information covered here is at an elementary level and is intended only to review or in some cases provide a first view of these very complicated topics. As a result, they are covered in a brief, simplified form. For a more detailed look at these processes and the cell itself, the student should refer to a cell biology textbook that covers cell structure, genetics, and protein synthesis.

Cells

Cells can be very different from each other. On a most basic level, we refer to cells as either *eukaryotic* or *prokaryotic*. Most of this textbook discusses the function of eukaryotic cells, which are found in animals and plants. Bacteria and other microorganisms are typically prokaryotic. The major

127

difference is that eukaryotic cells interact with one another to provide the metabolic activity required for a multicellular organism. Prokaryotic cells generally function by themselves to provide their own individual metabolic activity needed for that cell. The other major difference is that while eukaryotic cells have a defined nucleus, prokaryotic cells do not.

The nucleus is a good place to start this discussion, as it is the largest organelle, or component, of the eukaryotic cell and is a repository for deoxyribonucleic acid (DNA) and ribonucleic acid (RNA), substances responsible for protein synthesis. DNA is replicated (reproduced) here and transcribed to RNA. We discuss this process briefly later in this appendix.

The other components of cells are also important. For instance, while the cells of animals have a plasma membrane surrounding them, plant cells have a much more structured cell wall. Mitochondria are found in most cells, because they provide a location for transforming energy-yielding substances to usable forms of energy, like adenosine triphosphate (ATP). The endoplasmic reticulum provides a surface for the production of proteins on ribosomes as well as a conduit for the movement of synthesized materials from the cell to the outside of the cell. Several other organelles present in most cells are either involved in the transport of cell products, destruction of the cell when it is no longer useful, or destruction of materials that may reduce the cell's survival.

A multicelled organism, such as a plant, animal, or human, must have different cell types so that the organism can carry out its functions. For instance, in the animal or human, there is a need for red blood cells to carry oxygen from the lungs to the rest of the body. Mucosal cells of the digestive tract, respiratory tract, or the urinary tract must be capable of allowing, respectively, for the passage of food and absorption of nutrients, the passage of oxygen, and the passage of urine. In addition, these mucosal cells are also responsible for producing mucus, which acts not only as a lubricant but also as a barrier to infection. Other types of cells are used for our muscles, bones, and nervous systems. They are unique to their function and may have different structures in addition to producing different proteins from each other. All of these cells work in harmony—from the individual tissue to the organ to the entire organism—to ensure the sustenance of the human, animal, or plant.

Genetics and Protein Synthesis

As mentioned in the description of the cell, the nucleus is the site of DNA storage as well as its utility for protein synthesis. The DNA in the nucleus is a collection of chromosomes, each with specific components called *genes*.

Each gene has a specific, unique sequence of paired nucleotides forming a double helix, which looks something like a spiral staircase. The nucleotides in DNA are adenine, cytosine, guanine, and thymine. Although only four nucleotides are responsible for the structure of DNA, virtually an infinite number of combinations and sequences exist. Each of these genes, either by itself or coordinated with other genes, is responsible for producing a unique protein that is important either for the cell itself or to other organs and cells in the body that may receive it. The DNA is used to produce a template called RNA, which is a single strand of nucleotides. This strand is made up of mostly the same nucleotides, with the exception of uracil replacing thymine. The RNA, often referred to as *messenger RNA*, then attaches to the ribosomes. Amino acids are attached to each other by the action of another type of RNA, called *transfer RNA*, which enables specific amino acids to attach to each other to form a growing polypeptide chain. Ultimately these chains assemble into the specific proteins required for that individual, animal, or plant to thrive.

In fact, since the conclusion of the Human Genome Project earlier in this millennium, we now have a greater understanding about the uniqueness of protein synthesis in an individual. Although we only have a fractional knowledge about the importance of the various genes, we understand that people may express more or less of a particular protein as well as different proteins. This understanding has furthered our capacity to explain why we are all so very different. For instance, eye color is determined by several genes that may express proteins causing us to have blue, brown, green, or gold eyes. We have multiple genes that may express proteins causing us to have darker or lighter skin. Our heights, our gender, and our innate capacity for understanding are all influenced by our genes.

One of the more significant understandings is the contributions that small "errors" in the nucleotide sequence can make to result in disease or a higher probability of having a specific disease. The best example is the production of inappropriately shaped red blood cells. Sickle cell anemia is caused by just one mistake in the nucleotide sequence that would typically result in discoid-shaped red blood cells. The odd, sickle-shaped red blood cells that result from the defect cannot sufficiently transport oxygen to the body's cells, as discoid-shaped cells can do. Many diseases have been traced to a combination of single nucleotide errors, also known as *single nucleotide polymorphisms (SNPs)*, including cancers, heart disease, and diabetes. Much work remains to be done to understand these complex relationships, but progress is occurring at a great pace.

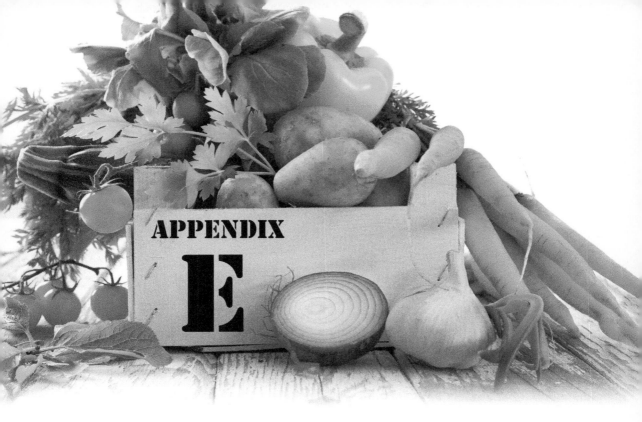

How Safe Is Our Food and Water Supply?

Although most of this book is dedicated to the nutrients available in our diets, the issue of the safety of our food supply is equally important. To fully understand the intricacies of the problems in providing food that is safe, a student would need to have a background in microbiology and chemistry and likely devote an entire semester to a course in food safety. This brief synopsis will attempt to provide insight into some of the issues and possible solutions to the problems. The issues that are faced include the possible microbiological contaminants and chemical additives and contaminants that may cause immediate or long-term consequences for a person eating certain foods or drinking particular beverages.

Microbes in our food supply can be either beneficial or detrimental. On the one hand, we know that the colonization of our colon by beneficial microbes enables the digestion of some fibers as well as promoting optimal function of the digestive system. These probiotics are usually found in designer foods like various yogurts or in capsular form. Although we are not entirely sure which microbes are the most beneficial, research studies are leading toward that direction. On the other hand, we have a very good knowledge of those microbes that may be found in some foods that cause adverse responses. These responses occur fairly quickly and are either due to the proliferation of the microbes themselves or to toxic substances that they produce.

There are an abundance of examples of these microbes, so first we discuss those that cause adverse responses in people due to their proliferation in the gastrointestinal tract. These infections are usually due to bacteria like Campylobacter, C. perfringens, E. coli, Listeria, or salmonella. Additionally, some infections are due to norovirus. The time from consumption to symptoms ranges from less than one day to up to about a week. Although these infections have different symptoms, the most common include diarrhea, vomiting, fever, and abdominal pain. In general, the presence of these microbes in foods is due to nonsanitary food handling, cooking foods inadequately, and a lack of proper refrigeration.

Other microbes and parasites produce toxic materials after ingestion. Those that are often responsible for illness include C. botulinum, S. aureus, and the Toxoplasma parasite. There is also a wide range from ingestion to the appearance of symptoms, ranging from less than a day up to several weeks. Many of the symptoms caused by these organisms' toxins result in effects upon the nervous and cardio-respiratory systems, in addition to gastrointestinal discomfort. Just as with the microbes that cause disease through infection, the intoxicating organisms are generally introduced through nonsanitary food handling, inadequately cooked foods, a lack of proper refrigeration, and additionally, poor canning methods, particularly resulting in growth of C. botulinum and the subsequent release of the botulinum toxin.

Although the food industry as well as governmental agencies responsible for the safety of our food supply have worked together to prevent large outbreaks of disease due to the bacteria, parasites, and viruses cited above, there have still been several serious outbreaks of disease due to E. coli, salmonella, and Listeria since 2006. Although we depend upon the food industry and the government to protect our food supply, we still must maintain an active role in protecting ourselves. As mentioned earlier, many of these organisms proliferate due to inadequate cooking and improper refrigeration. In addition, produce should be washed thoroughly. In particular, recent studies have shown that produce purchased from some farmers' markets has been handled with less than satisfactory sanitary practice. In addition, the sanitation in other countries may not be as carefully monitored, so we need to be concerned with foods arriving from abroad. The FDA as well as the USDA are as vigilant as possible given their limited resources to inspect food products from our country and other countries for microbial contamination, but we must be active in protecting ourselves through thorough washing of produce and cooking of meats.

Chemical contaminants and additives may arise in our food and drinking water in several different ways. Most common are the disposal of industrial waste products in bodies of water and the ground, contamination of animal feed, and chemicals added to our food, as well as those arising from the containers in which food is stored. Although we are currently more aware and do have better government oversight to diminish the presence of harmful contaminants and additives, many sources still concern us.

At this time, due to the combined efforts of the U.S. Environmental Protection Agency (EPA) and private industry, we have greatly curtailed the disposal of industrial waste products into our bodies of water and the ground. In the past, heavy metals like mercury, cadmium, and lead were disposed of in ways that would lead to appearance in our food supply. We still must be concerned about disposal that occurred in the past as well as current international disposal. Consequently, the EPA is active here in the United States, while governmental agencies in other countries also work to curtail the disposal of industrial waste products that could find their way into human or animal food or water. The organic product of mercury, methylmercury, continues to be a problem in our food supply. Although we generally think that specific large fish that are often not commonly consumed have high levels of mercury, we are now finding that tuna, which is a large fish commonly consumed, does have high levels of methylmercury. In particular, pregnant women should limit their consumption of canned tuna, as the methylmercury can have a profound negative impact upon the nervous systems of their unborn children.

Contamination of animal feed also continues to be a problem. Two contaminants in particular have been problematic: polybrominated biphenyls (PBBs) and polychlorinated biphenyls (PCBs). The people eating meat from animals with these contaminants have experienced nervous system disorders, and some men have developed infertility.

Pesticides have also been a continuous problem in our food supply. Both the EPA and the FDA monitor the use of pesticides in the United States. They determine what levels are acceptable and what pesticides can be used. The major problem is the produce from abroad that we consume. Unfortunately, many countries do not restrict pesticide use as well as we do. In fact, companies in the United States actually sell to other nations pesticides that have been banned here. Although government inspectors try to prevent the banned pesticides from returning to us, as well as preventing unacceptable levels of permitted pesticides in this produce, government resources are limited, and completely preventing the return of these pesticides from abroad is impossible. We need to be careful with produce: washing the skin, often peeling the skin, and cooking our fruits and vegetables to reduce our intake of pesticides. Some of the most common fruits and vegetables that are contaminated with high levels of pesticides include apples, peaches, potatoes, and strawberries.

The FDA is responsible for regulating food additives and monitoring those contaminants that arise from food storage. As such, the GRAS (generally recognized as safe) list of tentative additives to food was developed as a starting point in determining what the food industry could and could not add to food. These additives were determined to present a very minimal risk to individuals, particularly with regard to the development of cancer. Over the years, some materials on this list have been eliminated when shown to promote undue risk, while others have been added when they have been determined not to promote significant risk. As a result, a variety of food additives are used, including those that prevent microbial growth, like nitrites; antioxidants, like sulfites and ascorbic acid; coloring agents, like caramel and the carotenoid lycopene; as well as numerous natural and artificial flavors and olfactory agents.

As mentioned earlier, sometimes chemicals inadvertently appear in our food supply due to the way foods are stored or packaged. Typically, the contamination is due to the coating on the inside of cans and plastics used for storage. The most controversial issue at this time is determining the levels of bisphenol A, which seems to come from the plastic bottles used for storing beverages. More research is needed to make an informed decision as to the toxicity of this chemical and its passage into various liquids.

Most of us are concerned about drinking water, whether from public water systems, wells, or bottled water. Public water systems generally use chlorine to reduce microbes from our water. Although an admirable gesture, some researchers have found that chlorine may be injurious to some individuals. Some individuals are also concerned about the mineral content of their water, with hard water containing minerals like calcium. Other minerals that may be found in high levels are iron and copper from the plumbing used as conduits. Although these minerals may be beneficial in enhancing our nutrient intake, at very high levels iron and copper can both be detrimental. In addition, these minerals from water often produce rings around our drains of varying shades and result in damage to appliances like dishwashers and washing machines. Well water can be equally problematic. Often the content is highly variable between different wells, and if not chlorinated, can easily acquire microbial growth.

People have looked for alternatives, given the potential problems from public or private water systems. Most commonly, with respect to water entering the home, many have turned to water purification systems. Although some are effective in removing various microbes and others in removing various contaminants, in order to determine the appropriate purification system, the water entering the home should first be tested professionally. After that, the correct purification system can be purchased and installed.

Many people have focused on alternatives to drinking tap water. One alternative is to buy bottled drinking water. Unfortunately, there is no standardization for bottled water, and it may not be any different than tap water or could be superior; there is just no way to know. The other alternative has been to purchase filter systems that can be used to purify small amounts of water for drinking. The nature of these filters needs to be explored more fully, and just as with whole-home filters, the type of filtration used needs to align with the water being purified.

Glossary

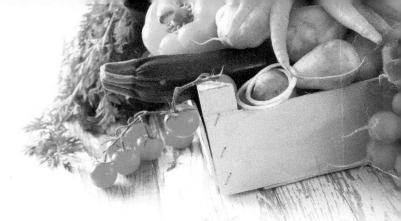

Adequate Intake (AI): Recommended amount of a nutrient based upon the average intake of healthy people of a specific age and gender.

Adipocytes: The technical name for fat cells, those cells that are biologically active in our adipose tissue that either store or release fat.

Amino acids: The building blocks of protein.

Anemia: A reduced level of red blood cells or a reduced functionality of the red blood cells.

Antioxidant: A chemical substance that reduces the capacity of other chemicals to result in oxidation of biological structures or materials.

Arrhythmias: A variety of disorders associated with the contractility of the heart, resulting in a beating pattern that is not associated with the normal action of the heart muscle. Often these take the form of irregularity of contractions or contractions that occur more rapidly than normal.

Atheromas: A mass of plaque consisting of various lipids and other cellular debris that generally obstructs blood flow in our arteries. Typically the cause of atherosclerosis.

Basal metabolic rate (BMR): The rate at which an individual uses energy irrespective of activity and other factors. It is usually dependent mostly on fat-free mass, gender, and age.

Bioavailablity: When referring to nutrients, the capacity of the gastrointestinal system to obtain a particular nutrient from food or pharmaceutical sources.

Calcitriol: The name used to refer to activated vitamin D, after it has been activated by the kidney and liver.

Cation: A positively charged ion found in the fluids of the body.

Collagen: A protein found in bone, joints, skin, and other areas in the body that provides flexibility to these areas due to the nature of the structure of this protein.

DEXA: An abbreviation for dual energy x-ray absorptiometry, a technique that can be used to measure bone density or body fat composition.

Dietary Recommended Intakes (DRIs): Nutrient intake values used in the United States and Canada, including the EARs, RDAs, AIs, EERs, and ULs.

Disaccharides: Simple sugars that are a combination of two monosaccharides. The most common ones found in food are sucrose, maltose, and lactose. In the human and animal body, the only one produced is lactose.

Diuretics: Medicines that encourage loss of body fluid; often used to reduce edema.

Diverticulitis: An infection of the colon, generally attributed to weak muscle walls, resulting in diverticulosis, followed by microorganisms entering the weakened areas, resulting in the infection.

Double-blind: An experimental design where neither the experimental nor control groups are aware of whether they are receiving a treatment and the investigators are also unaware of which subjects are in a treatment or control group.

Double bonds: The connection between some elements that are part of a molecule, which consists of two bonds between the elements, as compared to a single bond, which has only one connection. Double bonds are generally less stable to oxidation than single bonds.

Edema: Accumulation of fluid in the interstitial space, the area between our cells, and our vascular system. Usually results in a bloated appearance.

Eicosanoids: Biologically active molecules produced in the body from polyunsaturated fatty acids.

Endocrine: A term that refers to the organs of the system responsible for the release of hormones in the body.

Energy-yielding nutrient: A nutrient that can be broken down by the human body to be used for energy.

Enzymes: Specific proteins that are involved in either the breakdown, synthesis, or other types of transformation of a variety of molecules in our body.

Essential nutrient: A nutrient that people must consume to maintain health as they cannot either be made at all in the body or in adequate amounts to meet needs.

Estimated Average Requirements (EARs): The amount of a nutrient determined to meet the needs of healthy people of a specific age and gender.

Estimated Energy Requirements (EERs): The amount of energy determined to meet the needs of healthy people of a specific age and gender.

Exchange lists: Groups of food organized by their carbohydrate, protein, and fat composition used as a food-planning guide that can aid in weight control.

Fatty acids: Organic compounds that have a carbon chain, with one end being an inorganic acid and the other end being a methyl group.

Flavonoid: A chemical structure of numerous plant materials with a flavone component, many of which have biological activity.

Free radicals: Chemical substances that typically can attack DNA, RNA, and proteins, often damaging them so that they are no longer useful.

Fructose: A simple monosaccharide sugar, commonly found in fruits or as part of the table sugar (sucrose) molecule, sweeter than most other sugars.

Glucagon: A hormone released by the pancreas that results in the release of glucose from body stores of glycogen.

Glucose: A simple monosaccharide sugar, not usually found by itself, but part of all of the common disaccharides—including sucrose, mannose, and lactose—as well as the sugar that makes up starch chains.

Glycerol: The backbone of a triglyceride, composed of three carbons bonded together in a linear sequence, with each of the carbons having a hydroxyl group.

Glycogen: A storage form of glucose chains in the human and animal body, found as a branched-chain collection. Typically accumulates in muscles and liver.

Glycoproteins: Various proteins in the body that also contain sugar components. Some are very significant in ensuring that the other components of our bone, like hydroxyapatite and collagen, are held together properly.

Healthy Eating Index: A method primarily developed by the USDA to evaluate the quality of diets compared to recommendations.

Hematocrit: A measurement of the percentage of packed red blood cells as a part of the total blood volume.

Heme: The type of iron found in foods that is associated with either hemoglobin or similar molecules.

Hemoglobin: A protein produced in the body that uses iron to transport oxygen to tissues and cells that require oxygen.

High blood pressure (hypertension): A condition typified by having higher than normal blood pressure both when the heart is contracting to pump blood and also during the interval between the heart's contraction to pump the blood.

High-density lipoprotein (HDL): A lipoprotein particle produced in the liver that is low in cholesterol and high in specific proteins, capable of removing cholesterol from the body for disposal.

Hormone: A biologically active molecule produced in one part of the body that effects the activity of other cells or organs. Often, hormonelike molecules produced in the body may affect cells or organs in close proximity to the site of production.

Hydrolyzed: The action where parts of energy-yielding molecules are separated from other components with a resultant release of energy, which is typically how disaccharides and starches are broken down to monosaccharides.

Hydroxyapatite: A substance similar to that found in bone, composed of a matrix of calcium, phosphorus, and hydroxide ion. Typically, in the human body, there are numerous substitutions for these components, including fluoride and magnesium.

Initiation: When referring to tumors, the initial activity that results in the start of the growth of the tumor in a single cell.

Inorganic: A chemical substance containing neither a carbon-carbon or a carbon-hydrogen bond

Insulin: A hormone released by the pancreas that is extremely important in the proper uptake of glucose by many of the body's cells.

Intracellular water: The fluid contained within the various cells of the body.

Kwashiorkor: A nutritional disorder resulting from inadequate protein and calories and that causes edema, fatty liver, and other degenerative changes. It mostly occurs in young children.

Lipoprotein: A variety of different particles that are produced in the body that transport lipids, which also have specific proteins as part of them that result in either enhanced targeting of the lipoprotein to various tissues or organs or enhanced enzymatic activity associated with fat metabolism at a specific tissue or organ.

Low-density lipoprotein (LDL): A lipoprotein particle produced in the blood that is high in cholesterol and deposited in various organs as well as arteries.

Macrocytic: A cell that is smaller than comparable cells of that particular type. This term commonly refers to red blood cells that are smaller than typical red blood cells.

Marasmus: A nutritional disorder that results from inadequate protein and calories and causes poor growth and emaciation in children.

Megaloblastic: A cell that is typified by having an irregular structure. This term commonly refers to red blood cells that are not shaped in their typical ovular form.

Molecules: Compounds consisting of one or more atoms of at least one element.

Monoglycerides: Common name for a *monoacylglycerol*, a lipid with only one fatty acid esterified to a glycerol backbone.

Monosaccharides: Simple sugars that may either be available directly from foods or result from the breakdown of disaccharides or starches. The three major ones are glucose, fructose, and galactose.

Nonheme: The type of iron found in foods that is not associated with either hemoglobin or similar molecules. It constitutes the majority of iron found in most diets.

Nutrients: Chemical substances that supply energy or are used for maintenance, structure, or regulation.

Organic: A chemical substance containing either a carbon-carbon or a carbon-hydrogen bond.

Osteoporosis: A disorder occurring more commonly in women of advanced years that involves a reduced amount of bone. Often, osteoporosis leads to bone fractures due to the weakness of the bone.

Ostopenia: Reduction in the levels of bone compared to the normal healthy individual.

Phenolic: A chemical structure derived from phenol, an aromatic crystalline compound, often with biological activity.

Placebo: A substance provided to an individual that provides no health benefit but is comparable in taste and texture to a substance that may provide a specific health benefit.

Plaque: Often used similarly to the term *atheroma*, as they are collections of various lipids and cellular debris that accumulate on the intima of arteries.

Polyunsaturated fats: Fats generally found as liquids at room temperature and characterized by having fatty acids with two or more double bonds.

Prebiotic: A particular food substance that enhances the growth of microorganisms in the intestine, generally referring to microorganisms that improve digestion.

Propagation: When referring to tumors, the cellular events that result in continued growth of a tumor as many cells with the same expression.

Recommended Dietary Allowances (RDAs): The amount of a nutrient that has been determined to satisfy the nutritional needs of at least 98% of healthy individuals of a specific age and gender.

Red blood cells: Also known as erythrocytes, these cells carry hemoglobin, which results in their red color. They are critical as an oxygen delivery system to the body's cells.

Solubility: The extent to which a particular chemical can be dissolved in a specific solvent.

Solvents: A liquid substance that can be used for dissolving another substance.

Starches: Various collections of glucose molecules in large chains; some may be linear where others may be branched. Generally each plant food has its own particular starch.

Sterols: Organic compounds that have a specific four-ring carbon structure.

Subcutaneous: Below the skin.

Sugars: Simple carbohydrates, including monosaccharides and disaccharides.

Tetany: An uncontrollable twitching of a muscle, often due to mineral imbalance.

Tolerable Upper Intake (UL): The highest amount of a nutrient that can be safely consumed without adverse health effects for an individual of a specific age and gender.

Trans-monounsaturated fat: A type of fatty acid, sometimes found in nature, but occurring in high amounts after polyunsaturated oils have been treated chemically to result in monounsaturated fat. The fatty acids have a trans configuration around the remaining double bond, meaning that the hydrogen atoms of the two adjacent carbon structures are on the opposite sides.

Transamination: A biochemical process whereby an amino group from a particular amino acid is transferred to a ketoacid, resulting in a new nonessential amino acid and a new ketoacid.

Triglycerides: Common name for the chemical compound also known as a *triacylglycerol*. It is composed of a glycerol backbone, where each of the hydroxyl groups is esterified with a fatty acid.

Vasodilation: Expansion of the vessels of the circulatory system to allow for greater volumes of blood passage through them.

Vegan: An individual who refrains from consuming animal meats as well as the products of animals such as eggs and milk products.

About the Author

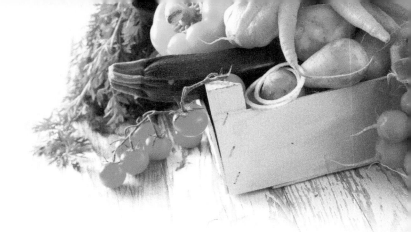

Dr. Leonard E. Gerber received his undergraduate training at Columbia University and his doctoral training at the University of Illinois at Urbana-Champaign. After receiving his Ph.D. in nutrition, he spent two years doing postdoctoral work at the University of Illinois, focusing on nutrition and wound healing. Since 1981 he has been a faculty member in the Department of Nutrition and Food Sciences at the University of Rhode Island. In addition to teaching an introductory course in nutrition, he also teaches an undergraduate course in micronutrients and a graduate course in vitamins and minerals. Dr. Gerber has had a distinguished record of service at the university, including director of research compliance, chair of the Institutional Review Board for Human Subject Use, and chair of the Institutional Animal Care and Use Committee. He serves on the editorial board for several nutrition journals and the Advisory Board for Annual Editions: Nutrition. He has also served as an ad-hoc reviewer for several other nutrition journals, including *Nutrition and Cancer: An International Journal*. Dr. Gerber has written numerous publications in the field of nutrition and presented many abstracts at scientific meetings. He has been a member of the American Society for Nutrition since 1979 and a member of the Vitamins and Minerals Interest Group and Diet and Cancer Interest Group of the ASN since 2007.

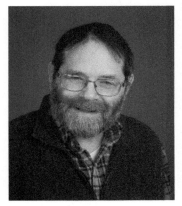

Dr. Leonard E. Gerber

His current research focuses mainly on the impact and role of vitamin E and similar compounds. In addition, Dr. Gerber also is interested in exploring the possible relationships between diet and autism.

Index

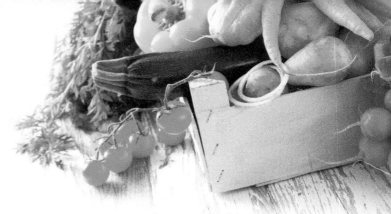